O WHAT A
TANGLED WEB

MONICA BLAND

O what a tangled web we weave
When first we practise to deceive!
Sir Walter Scott

First published in Great Britain by
Pen Press Publishers Ltd
25 Eastern Place
Brighton
BN2 1GJ

ISBN13: 978-1-906206-73-4

Printed and bound in Great Britain by
Cpod, Trowbridge, Wiltshire

A catalogue record of this book is available from
the British Library

Cover design by Jacqueline Abromeit

Sometimes the most ordinary people can have their quiet and routine lives disrupted by the most extraordinary and unexpected events. Monica Bland was one such person. Looking forward to a peaceful but active retirement with her husband, she was suddenly struck down with serious illness. She found herself not only having to deal with a life-threatening condition, but also with the strong likelihood that she was the victim of a medical cover-up. This is her true story, told in her own words, of her long struggle for truth and justice.

The names of people and places have been changed to conceal true identities.

CHAPTER 1

"To begin at the beginning."

The 31st of May 1981 was a Saturday. Back in those days when I worked full-time as a lecturer in a further education college, Saturday was a day for catching up on housework, doing some gardening, and going out. It was my favourite day of the week. I woke up feeling relaxed, planning my day, and looking forward to the Yetties concert at the Casterbridge Arts Centre my husband, Mike, and I would attend in the evening.

But something was wrong. I'd got that nagging abdominal pain again. I got up, telling myself that once I got moving, had had some breakfast and gone to the loo, it would go, as it had before. It was probably wind. This time the pain got worse. I staggered down to breakfast, but half way through my cornflakes I went back up to bed, hoping a quiet lie-down would help.

Mike followed me up. Something must have indicated to him that things were serious. He almost dragged me out of bed, bundled me into the car, and took me to the doctor's surgery. Back in 1981 most GPs still held Saturday morning surgeries.

Dr Moore was an elderly GP, a man of great wisdom and perception, according to Mike, but of few words. I hardly knew him, as being a healthy woman, I'd only visited him once or twice. He soon had me on the couch, examining my bare abdomen with his cold hands, but not saying anything. To my horror, he insisted on having a poke up my vagina as well. Whether this enlightened him further, I don't know.

"So what's the problem?" I asked, doing up my trousers and sitting down by his desk.

"Can't say. Could be wind or a bowel upset, or something more serious. Take these pain killers." He thrust some drug company freebies over the desk. "If you still have pain by this evening, contact the duty doctor."

By early evening I was still in pain. Mike took me to see a Dr Snow, who happened to have drawn the short straw that weekend. He also happened to be the worst GP in town. Terrible stories about him circulated around the hairdressers. So it was up on the couch again for more abdominal pummelling accompanied this time by a rectal prod.

"You have appendicitis," he announced with great authority.

"Are you sure?" I asked.

"Quite sure. You will need an operation. I'll arrange for your immediate admission to hospital." He picked up the phone and contacted the admissions office.

I tried to collect my thoughts. "How long will I be off work?" I asked.

"About a month."

Things could be worse. I was relieved that it was just appendicitis. I'd have a routine operation, a week in hospital, and three weeks lying in the sun. My work at the college was almost over for the year – public exams started in a week or two, and what the students didn't know now, they'd never know. There would be some internal exams to set and mark, and reports to write, but I could do all that at home. Mike also worked at the college, so he'd be able to ferry papers back and forth. I'd earn my sick pay.

We returned home, collected a few things, and drove to Casterbridge General Hospital. As we approached the imposing modern building, doubts began to build up in my mind. I voiced them to Mike.

"I've had this pain before. It always comes midway between

my periods. Perhaps it's something gynaecological, something to do with ovulation."

"You'd better tell the doctors about it," Mike replied curtly. He didn't like discussing 'women's problems'.

Even back in 1981 it was best to arrange to fall ill between 9am and 5pm on a weekday. 7pm on a Saturday is not the best time to be admitted to a hospital with a possibly inaccurate diagnosis. The consultants are all mooring their yachts, or wandering in from the golf course, and booking tables at fancy restaurants. Meanwhile their juniors hold the fort, working ridiculous hours, almost dead on their feet.

A number of these poor souls came and prodded me, fortunately not internally. I told them all about my gynaecological theories, but only a lady doctor seemed prepared to listen, and even she stuck to the appendicitis verdict, along with all her male colleagues. I was firmly labelled as 'the appendix in bed 14'.

I had a disturbed night. The pain got worse, and was only bearable if I stayed sitting up. Sleeplessness only increased my doubts and fears. Why were the doctors so dismissive of my own views and intimate knowledge of my own body? If a pain only occurred periodically, surely it was reasonable to suspect it was linked to what went on periodically – i.e. ovulation. But I had to remind myself that I wasn't a doctor. I'd had no medical training whatsoever. My degree was in geography. I knew the layout of the world, but was a little hazy about the layout of my internal organs. I had to trust the doctors. I was in a good modern hospital. They knew what they were doing. Yet the anxieties remained.

Sunday morning dawned at last. I wasn't allowed breakfast, not that I felt like any. There was more pressing and prodding of my abdomen. The diagnosis remained the same. The doctors wanted to operate right away. Consent forms for an appendectomy were thrust in front of me.

"I'm not sure it is appendicitis," I told them. "I want to phone my husband before I sign."

I poured out all my fears to Mike on the phone in the day room.

"But something's got to be done," he said, sounding rather exasperated.

"I don't want to be cut open if it's not necessary," I replied quite reasonably.

"Look, you're in pain. Something's seriously wrong. It's got to be seen to. If it isn't your appendix, they'll find out what it is and hopefully put it right."

"But I'm just consenting to an appendectomy. They can't do anything else."

"They can if it's for your own good. You've just got to trust them."

Mike was right. Eventually I signed the form, but I added under 'appendectomy', 'anything else that needs to be done'.

I was wheeled off to the operating theatre that afternoon. It was scary. I'd never had an operation or general anaesthetic before. The anaesthetist got to work and I drifted into unconsciousness.

Two hours later I woke up back in the ward. Mike was sitting by my bed. He looked as white as a sheet. He slipped my watch back on my wrist, as he knew I always liked to know the time. My throat was sore, and I didn't want to talk. Yet already a question had formed in my slightly befuddled mind. Did appendectomies take two hours? Weren't they quick, simple operations? Perhaps I'd just been asleep for a long time afterwards. I didn't want to know anything. I just wanted to sleep.

Next morning a nurse came to wash me. I saw the dressing on a diagonal wound on the right side of my abdomen.

"Was it my appendix?" I asked.

"No. They removed your right ovary. It was a cyst, I think. We'll be transferring you to the gynae ward."

The news came as no great surprise. In fact, I experienced a small frisson of satisfaction that I had proved the doctors wrong. I contemplated saying "told you so" when they came on their round, but wisely thought the better of it. I was in their hands. I didn't want to antagonise them.

Later that day I was wheeled through the gleaming corridors to the gynaecological ward, and Mike came in. It appeared he had been in the hospital while the operation was going on, and the surgeon had briefed him thoroughly.

"It was a growth," he said. "The left ovary is also affected. You may need another op."

Growth? Cyst? What was the difference? Somehow 'growth' sounded more sinister.

"Why didn't they remove both ovaries?" I asked. "I'd given permission."

"They'd never do that – not to a childless fertile woman of thirty-five. You'd have been able to sue them."

"But we don't want kids."

"They weren't to know that."

At long last I managed to steel myself to ask the question which had been nagging away at the back of my mind since Saturday.

"It's not cancer, is it?"

"Everything was sent to the pathology lab for tests. It'll take a few days, I'm afraid." Mike seemed nervy. Did he know more than he was letting on? Or was it just understandable anxiety?

During the next few days doctors kept asking me if I wanted children. I was quite adamant that I didn't, but they didn't seem to believe me. I kept asking the doctors if it was cancer.

"Most unlikely in a woman of your age," was the comforting reply. I did believe them this time. I wanted to. Only old people got cancer, I told myself.

What was very noticeable was the total absence of any kind of apology. They had got it wrong and they knew it. There was not a hint of contrition. Had they explained that appendicitis and ovarian problems on the right side could be confused, and that in my case they had unfortunately made an inaccurate diagnosis, I might have been more favourably disposed towards them. But no, nothing was forthcoming. As I was to learn over the years, doctors never admit that they can be wrong.

On the Friday morning I was given the news that the pathology lab had indeed found cancer cells. It was ovarian cancer. The doctors seemed almost as distressed as I was. It was so unusual in one so young. I phoned Mike at the college, and he came straight to the hospital. Already future treatment was being discussed. There seemed to be more concern about preserving my fertility than tackling the dreaded disease. Mike made it quite clear to the consultant that neither of us wanted children. It was therefore decided that radiotherapy would be a better treatment than chemotherapy. I was relieved. All I could think about was that chemotherapy made your hair fall out and that almost seemed a fate worse than death. Perhaps it was a pity that nobody had told me that it soon grows again.

Casterbridge General Hospital swung into action with a speed I didn't know existed in the NHS. I saw Dr Carson, the radiologist, that very day. He answered all my questions about radiotherapy, and without making any rash promises, assured me that the treatment would be highly effective against my early stage cancer. The downside was that my periods would cease and that I would be infertile. For me, it wasn't a problem. In fact, it would be great to be rid of periods. He commented on how young I was, which he said was very much in my favour. He had only had one case of someone younger than me. I felt he had an unusual level of professional interest in me, and that was good.

But what had caused the cancer? I had a reasonably healthy lifestyle. I'd never smoked, I hardly ever drank alcohol, and I ate a balanced diet. I was slightly overweight, but not by enough to affect my health. At the time my activities in the Campaign for Nuclear Disarmament had made me acutely aware of the dangers of radiation. What can cure can also kill in the wrong doses. It seemed that radiation had a particularly adverse effect on the reproductive organs. Recuperating in hospital, I had plenty of time to ponder matters. What about the Windscale fire of 1957? A plume of radioactive particles had drifted as far south as Kent, where I had been living at the time, and where, at the age of eleven, my ovaries would have been gearing up for action. Then what about the radioactive material used for experiments in the laboratory where my father worked? My sister and I used to play in the corridors around the labs if my father was on duty at weekends. There was a pit in a nearby orchard where they dumped radioactive material, and where we weren't allowed to go. We dared each other to approach it, as kids do. What about the watch with luminous hands I'd worn non-stop for years? Once in a physics lesson at school, I'd put it near a Geiger counter. The machine went mad. I thought it was fun at the time. What about those X-ray machines they used to have in shoe shops? I just loved seeing the bones in my toes wriggling in the strange green light. I insisted on having a go every time I had new shoes. I thought it was fun at the time.

Why had I been struck down when so young? Women in their thirties just didn't get ovarian cancer – Dr Carson had made that clear. I became increasingly convinced that the cause of my cancer was environmental, but that I would never know exactly what had caused it. I just had to accept the situation and concentrate on getting better. A positive mental attitude was vital.

Three weeks after my operation I started on a ten-week course of radiotherapy. Every weekday I went to the hospital and lay on the narrow stretcher while the big radiotherapy machine circled round me, zapping me from above and below. I willed the rays to do their stuff.

I was advised not to rush back to the hurly-burly of college life, and didn't return until November. I went to Dr Moore for my sick certificates.

"It was a bit of a shock it turned out to be cancer," I commented one day.

He looked at me with his tired, wise eyes. "I thought it was cancer," he said. He didn't elaborate, and I didn't know what to say.

Regular check-ups with Dr Carson went on for years, at first three-monthly, then six-monthly, then annually. In February 1987 he proclaimed me cured.

I was, of course, grateful that the NHS and modern medicine had cured me, but the whole episode had left me with a deeply seated mistrust of doctors. Perhaps the outcome would have been better if the doctors had listened to me. Perhaps then I would have been operated on by a gynaecologist with experience of pelvic cancers. He, or she, might have realised that the left ovary should also have been removed. Who could tell whether or not I was cured? Perhaps there was a time-bomb ticking inside me.

CHAPTER 2

I stayed well. In 1983 Mike and I, becoming increasingly disillusioned with education, left the college and set up an accountancy practice. Mike was a Chartered Accountant. He did all the clever work, and I did all the donkey work. We did well. Over the years the practice expanded and we took on staff. I continued to work part-time, mainly looking after the practice finances, a task Mike preferred not to farm out to employees.

I usually worked at home rather than at the office. Commuting for me was walking from the kitchen to my desk in the lounge, visiting the loo on the way. On the 18th of December 1999, a Friday, I never made it to the lounge because something happened in the loo.

There was a smear of dark red blood on the toilet tissue. Where on earth had that come from? There were three possible sources. I probed carefully. It was coming from my vagina. A cold shiver went through me. After over eighteen years, the cancer was back, I thought. Or was it? Perhaps I was jumping to unwarranted conclusions. A number of things could cause vaginal bleeding. I even wondered whether, at the age of fifty-three I was starting my periods again. Did anyone know about the long-term effects of radiotherapy? Had my remaining left ovary sprung back into action after a long period of dormancy? If it was very rare to get cancer and have radiotherapy at thirty-five, there would be very few people alive eighteen years after a course of radiotherapy. Old age and other diseases would have despatched patients who had been diagnosed in their fifties and sixties, unless the cancer had got them first.

This was all pointless speculation. I had to contact the doctor right away. I went into the hall and phoned the surgery. Despite explaining the nature of my problem, and my understandable anxiety, I couldn't get an appointment until the following Monday evening. Over the weekend I did my best to cope with my fears by joking with my menopausal contemporaries that I was starting my periods. I also thought about other things. Had I been ignoring warning signs that my health was deteriorating? For the last few weeks I'd been feeling tired. I'd put it down to prolonged jet-lag after our holiday in New Zealand followed by having to hit the ground running on my return to catch up on the backlog of work after a month away. I was also suffering from a persistent but mild sore throat. Then there were the tender nipples, just like I used to have before a period. What was going on?

Dr Moore had retired in the early 1980s and his practice had been taken over by Dr Peter Foyle and his partners. Over the years, on my rare visits to the surgery, I would see whoever happened to be available, and on the Monday evening this happened to be Dr Foyle. I ran through all my strange symptoms, and I soon found myself up on the couch without my trousers and briefs. Dr Foyle felt my abdomen, commenting that it seemed unusually large. I thought it was just middle-age spread. He then gave me the most brutal vaginal examination I had ever had. When I complained about how much he was hurting me he said I was making too much fuss. At last he withdrew his gloved finger. It was dripping with fresh red blood.

"Oh yes, you are bleeding," he remarked. It was quite different to the small amounts of dark blood I had noticed, and I suspected his examination had caused the bleeding. But I didn't say anything. Perhaps I should have done.

I got dressed and sat down by his desk again.

"I think you have a cyst," he said.

"Do you think it's cancer?" I asked.

"Could be. In view of your previous history I'll fast-track you to Ellman or one of the other gynae boys at the hospital. You'll get an appointment within two weeks."

I knew I was in for a miserable Christmas. The 'could be cancer' diagnosis would hang over me throughout the festive season. How could I possibly be jolly and full of seasonal cheer? Somehow I got through the office dinner the following evening, and fortunately, preferring a quiet life, Mike and I had very few social engagements. I developed bouts of trembling accompanied by sweating from my hands and feet. Was this anxiety or another strange symptom with a physical cause? By Boxing Day I was in such a state I decided to see the emergency doctor. After a two-hour wait, a hurried consultation with an obviously weary doctor resulted in him diagnosing depression and prescribing an anti-depressant. He had not carried out any physical examination, not even checking my pulse and temperature. I just couldn't believe it. I was convinced my symptoms were physical in origin. Over the years I had had my fair share of stress, but I had never before experienced the symptoms I now had. I didn't collect the anti-depressant. Instead I popped the prescription, along with a note of explanation to Dr Foyle, through the surgery door. Once he was functioning again after Christmas he phoned me, agreeing that I did not need anti-depressants.

Because of the Christmas period, the two-week fast-track stretched to three weeks. On the 10th of January 2000 I saw Ellman's registrar. After more uncomfortable examinations, he ordered an urgent ultrasound scan. The 'could be cancer' diagnosis remained. No attention at all was paid to all my other symptoms. Nothing seemed to have changed since 1981. The doctors still wouldn't listen to me. All my mistrust started to surface again.

The following week I received the results of the scan. It appeared that the mass, although large, was filled with fluid and unlikely to be cancerous. There was slight concern about something in the uterus. The registrar told me I would need the cyst and left ovary removed, and a hysterectomy. Although the news was better than it could have been, I still faced a serious operation. Was it really necessary? Could the cyst be drained? Had adequate tests been done? Things seemed a bit slip-shod, and I hadn't had a chance to discuss things with the consultant. I decided to write to him describing my various symptoms. At least then he could not plead ignorance if there were any cock-ups.

Because cancer could not be ruled out, the operation was booked for the 1st of February. On 31 January I was admitted and had to wait in the day room for a bed to be prepared. Suddenly a large entourage around a file trolley appeared in the doorway. A tall, dark, but not particularly handsome man appeared to be in charge.

"This is Monica Bland," one of his minions told him, handing him a file. He quickly glanced inside it, and then looked at me.

"Hello, Mrs Bland. We haven't met before, have we? I'm Mr Ellman. Are you happy about your operation tomorrow?"

Arrogance oozed from every pore on his skin. His entourage of nurses and junior doctors seemed ill-at-ease, almost cringing in his presence. I took an instant dislike to the man, something which was extremely rare for me. I suppose he was expecting the usual humble "yes, thank you" reply to his question. He seemed to physically recoil when I answered, "No. Didn't you get my letter about my symptoms and concerns?"

He looked taken aback, although his body language struck me as rather theatrical.

"I've not seen any letter. I'll ask my secretary about it".

"I sent it over a week ago."

He started moving along the corridor, obviously not

wishing to give me any more time. A member of his entourage broke away and stayed with me, somewhat furtively, I thought.

"I'm Natalie Yeo. I'm one of the nurses on Mr Ellman's team. What's worrying you?"

She spent some time with me while I poured out my concerns. She listened, and for that I was grateful. But she made no comments, and I doubted whether she would have any influence on Ellman, or even that she would have a chance to convey my worries. I didn't want to create chaos by cancelling the operation at the last minute, so things went ahead as planned.

The day after the operation Mr Ellman saw me and explained that he had removed the cyst along with my left ovary and Fallopian tube. He had also performed a sub-total hysterectomy which meant I still had my cervix. Some material looked suspicious, and he could not rule out cancer until the pathology results were available, but he was ninety-nine per cent sure he had removed everything that needed removing. I smiled to myself at the 'ninety-nine per cent'. Really it meant he was completely confident that he had done a satisfactory job, but as nothing can be certain in medicine, he had covered himself. Doctors had to be so careful in these litigious times, I thought. I still couldn't stand the man. He still struck me as arrogant and distant, and this time, strangely nervous. I told myself it didn't really matter what I thought of him, just so long as he'd done a decent job on my insides. I'd probably never see him again.

Later that week I saw Natalie Yeo again. It turned out she was a Macmillan nurse, a specialist in cancer care. She talked to me about chemotherapy. I was worried. Although the pathology results were not available, it seemed she was preparing me for the worst. She sat on my bed, appearing thin and washed out. She yawned. It must be the emotional strain of her job, I thought. I knew I wouldn't be able to do it, and I greatly admired her. All the same, from then on I referred to her as the drippy Natalie.

17

Eight days after the operation I was able to leave hospital. The pathology results were still not available. How I coped, I don't know. In 1981 I had the results after five days. Why were things taking so much longer in 2000? Movement was still causing me considerable pain and I was concerned that my recovery seemed much slower than after my previous operation. But now I was nineteen years older, and I had had more done. I would just have to take things easy for a few weeks.

I finally received the pathology results after a three-week wait. How could it have taken so long? It was inhuman. A rather ambiguous letter from Ellman explained that some cells had shown borderline changes, but that he was confident that there was little chance of further disease, and that no further treatment was necessary. I would have a check-up at six weeks after the operation, and that, it appeared, would be the end of the matter. I breathed an enormous sigh of relief. It seemed things had been caught in the nick of time. Once more I had cheated the big C. I felt invincible.

The hysterectomy recovery notes I had been given said that after six weeks I should be able to walk for forty-five minutes without pain or tiredness. I felt a total wreck after five minutes. Shopping was absolutely exhausting. Then there was the unexpected vaginal discharge, which appeared a month after the operation. I went to the doctor's about it, seeing Dr Green, one of the partners. She was concerned, and contacted Mr Ellman. According to him it was normal – strange the recovery notes didn't mention it. Around the middle of March, as I gradually became more active, I developed bowel problems, constantly passing mucus and rabbit droppings. Over the next two months, despite six visits to the doctor and various medicines for both diarrhoea and constipation, I was no better. I saw Dr Foyle early in May. He told me he thought the problem was 'something mechanical' but that it was nothing to worry about. I took the term 'mechanical' to mean that it was something to do with the configuration of the bowel, which might have been disturbed by the operation. I was to have an ultrasound scan at the end of August, and it seemed he thought there was no reason to bring this forward. I instinctively knew there was something wrong but, once more, no one would listen.

I consulted an old friend, Terry Sutton, a homeopath. I had a completely open mind about the effectiveness of homeopathy, but seeing conventional medicine was failing me, it was worth a try. Among other investigations and treatments, Terry tried out a new diagnostic tool on me. It measured external and internal body temperature, the theory being that cancers were hotter than normal tissue. Results showed a big hot spot low down in my pelvis, but the problem was that this could be due to post-operative inflammation. It was all very confusing for me. I soldiered on, hoping my bowels would slowly return to normal.

CHAPTER 3

At my six-week check-up, despite the assurances I had received in Ellman's letter, the member of his team that I saw had been instructed that I would need further scans and check-ups. Perhaps the cancer threat was more serious than Ellman had led me to believe. I was going to have to learn to live in a constant state of uncertainty which was not helped by what appeared to be frequent changes of mind by the doctors.

On the 10th of September 2000 I had an appointment to get the result of my recent ultrasound scan. Fortunately I didn't see Ellman, instead seeing his registrar, Dr Hick, an Australian lady who seemed strangely ill-at-ease. But then everyone on Ellman's team seemed ill-at-ease.

"How do you feel?" she asked.

"Quite well except for some bowel problems, but they seem to be slowly improving."

She looked down at the scan report. "I'm afraid the scan shows another mass has formed."

I looked at her in stunned silence. So much for 'little chance of further disease'. I wanted the facts, however unpalatable they might be.

"Where is it?"

"Low down in the pelvis, just above the cervix."

"How big is it?"

Dr Hick formed her hands into a sphere about the size of a grapefruit. Goodness, it was huge, but that did suggest it was a cyst rather than a cancerous tumour.

"Is it cancer?"

"We don't know, but you will need a further operation. These things happen, I'm afraid."

What things, I wondered. The formation of further cysts? Then I remembered the blood test I'd had at the time of the scan. It was called a CA125 test and measured something in the blood which could indicate the presence of ovarian cancer. In January it had been slightly raised, but not high enough to worry the doctors unduly. It was explained to me that certain other infections could cause it to rise. It didn't strike me as a very reliable test. All the same, I still wanted the result.

"What about the CA125 blood test?"

Dr Hick looked through the papers in my file. "It's just above normal and considerably lower than in January, but we can't totally rely on it."

Dr Hick asked a nurse to take me to the admissions office. It seemed she wanted to move fast. With amazing efficiency I was given an operation date in ten day's time. I got the feeling they were worried about me. Without much hope of getting one at such short notice, I asked for an amenity bed. It was a scheme whereby I could pay for a side room for peace and quiet while still receiving free NHS care. I had had one in February, and I think it had helped with my recovery.

On the 20th of September I was once more admitted to Casterbridge General Hospital. To my surprise and delight I was shown straight to a perfectly prepared side room with a beautiful distant sea view. It seemed extreme good fortune that such a lovely room had suddenly become available, almost too good to be true. However, I was beginning to get to the stage where if things seemed to be going too well, I became suspicious.

During the afternoon various junior doctors came to see me to check odd details. One said, "You have ovarian cancer."

"No," I corrected him. "I *had* ovarian cancer back in '81. They only found borderline cell changes last February."

The poor lad shuffled through my file, looking confused. He's just a bit wet behind the ears, I thought. Perhaps someone had briefed him on my history and he had misheard 'had' for 'have'. It was an easy mistake to make. I didn't think any more of it.

The following morning I found I was third on the list to go to the operating theatre. This struck me as a little odd. The scan could only show so much, and a subsequent sigmoidoscopy – a peep up the rectum with a camera on a flexible tube – had shown that the cyst was probably attached to the bowel. It was possible that a small section of bowel might have to be removed, and my agreement to this had been obtained. It could turn out to be a complicated operation. Ellman, who I presumed would be performing the operation, would be less than fresh, and probably thinking more about his lunch than about me.

I wasn't actually wheeled into the operating theatre until midday. I knew nothing more until I woke up about one and a half hours later back in my room. The time scale suggested nothing too serious had been done, although I was attached to all the usual tubes and dips. A few minutes later Mike appeared, looking grim.

"What did they do?" I asked.

"Nothing."

"Nothing! What the hell's going on?" Suddenly I was wide awake. I'd been cut open again from my navel to my groin for no good reason.

Mike tried to calm me. "I asked the nurse just now what you'd had done. She said didn't I know, so I said 'not exactly'. She looked at your notes and said 'nothing'. I couldn't believe it myself, but anyway, the doctor will see you soon and explain things."

"I'm a cut and shut, a hopeless case," I wailed. "They can't do anything."

"Don't jump to conclusions. Just be patient and wait until you've seen the doctor."

I flopped back on to the pillows and closed my eyes. I was riddled with cancer, I thought. But how come I was so well apart from the bowel problem? If you had advanced cancer you were meant to be tired and weak, and suffering from lack of appetite and weight loss. That's what it said in my medical encyclopedia – one of the more frequently thumbed books on my shelf. I was eating like a horse, as usual, very overweight, as ever, and bursting with energy. On the face of it, there seemed to be nothing wrong with me.

Mike stayed around, but we had to wait nearly four hours before the doctor came. Around six o'clock Dr Hick strode in, looking uncomfortable and self-conscious, as if she knew she was about to do something very unpleasant.

"The mass was close to major nerves and blood vessels," she explained in her strong Australian twang. "It was too dangerous to try and remove it, so we'll have to think about how else we can treat it. But it's not a nasty cancer." She paused and met my eyes. I got the strange feeling that her lips were saying one thing and her eyes something completely different. Her behaviour struck me as very odd. "We'll arrange for an MRI scan, and chemotherapy, if appropriate."

With that she was gone. I glanced at Mike. "What did you make of that?" I remarked. "She's acting strange."

Mike shrugged, lost for words. By now I was well over the anaesthetic and feeling quite perky. The brain went into overdrive. I had lived and worked in Australia for over six months during world travels in my twenties. I liked the Aussies. They were always direct and open, occasionally to the point of rudeness. They hadn't much time for the innuendoes or strange social codes of the prissy poms. You knew where you were with an Aussie. Yet I felt that Dr Hick was concealing something. It was as if she had been asked to do something which went completely against both her personal and professional ethical code, and she was making a right hash of it, perhaps deliberately, to alert me to something. But what? I just couldn't fathom it out, possibly because I was still a little woozy after the operation. Tomorrow was the time to give it all more thought.

"Oh, I nearly forgot," Mike said. "This came in the post this morning." He pulled a letter from his jacket pocket. It was from the hospital and contained notification of an appointment for some kind of test on my water works. I remembered that Dr Hick had ordered the test at our consultation. I had asked when I would have it when I attended for the pre-op checks, and had been told by a junior doctor that the test had not been considered necessary after all. So how come I had now received an appointment for this pre-op test on a date two weeks after the date of the operation?

"This is crazy," I fumed. "I'm in a mad-house. Nobody knows what they're doing"

Mike tried to calm me. "I expect they just forgot to cancel the request for a test."

"But it shouldn't happen," I went on. "There's no system. Everything seems so confused." I was almost in tears. Perhaps it was a minor cock-up with a simple explanation, but to me it was indicative of an organisation in chaos, possibly with life-threatening consequences.

That night I hardly slept at all. Everything swirled around in my head as the hands of the clock above the door crept through the small hours. 'Not a nasty cancer' Dr Hick had said. I suddenly realised what an ambiguous statement that was. For a lay person, every cancer is nasty, even tiny, easily curable ones. There could be no such thing as a 'nice' cancer. Therefore the words 'nasty' and 'cancer' naturally went together. 'Not a nasty cancer' therefore meant 'not a cancer'. The 'nasty' was redundant. But why had Dr Hick then talked about further treatment, MRI scans, and chemotherapy? That would suggest it was cancer. Perhaps 'not nasty' was relevant.

It probably meant it was a confined and curable cancer. Either way, things didn't seem too bleak. No doubt the situation would be clearer once the pathology reports came through. Then another thought struck me. If they hadn't removed anything, nothing would have gone to the lab. But surely they would have done a biopsy on the mass. Dr Hick hadn't mentioned that, as far as I could remember. I'd ask about it next time I saw her. At last I fell into a fitful doze until being woken at some uncivilised hour by a nurse taking my blood pressure.

Dr Hick came to see me again at about 6 pm. She asked me to repeat to her what she had told me the previous evening. I did so with complete accuracy, I believe, and joked that even though it had only been a few hours after the operation, I had been totally alert mentally. I expressed my concerns about the cancer uncertainties.

"I suppose I'll just have to be patient and wait for the pathology results on the biopsy," I said.

"I'm afraid we weren't able to get a biopsy," Dr Hick replied. "We tried, but it caused heavy bleeding, which wasn't very good for you. But we're testing some peritoneal fluid – fluid from the lining around your organs. That will show if there are any cancer cells around."

Once more I was aware of the strange way in which Dr Hick was looking at me, as if trying to convey something through her pale blue eyes. It was unnerving and confusing.

So, no biopsy, I mused after she had gone. It seemed odd. What if taking one had caused bleeding? I was lying in a state-of-the-art operating theatre. Bleeding is the norm when you're being cut open. They have efficient ways of controlling it. I would have thought that the importance of obtaining a biopsy would have far outweighed the need to prevent bleeding. But I wasn't a surgeon. I knew nothing about operating procedures, and didn't want to know. I had to trust the experts. There was no alternative.

It occurred to me that although Mr Ellman had performed the operation (assisted by Dr Hick) he had not put in an appearance. I was quite relieved, as I couldn't stand the man. Dr Hick, his registrar, and the junior doctors were providing perfectly adequate care. All the same, I did get the slight feeling that Mr Ellman was deliberately avoiding me.

Next morning Dr Hick visited me yet again. She explained that she was on Saturday duty in the maternity department. It seemed more a social call than anything. I felt quite sorry for her. It was the perfect late September day, and we both gazed longingly at the sparkling sea in the distance. Then, once more, her gaze turned on me. She wanted to tell me something, I just knew it. It was a woman-to-woman intuition thing. But then she was gone, striding off to deliver babies.

Rita, a good friend from the Scrabble club I belong to, came in that afternoon with her board and tiles to cheer me up with a game. But first she had to listen to all my woes. She frowned and tut-tutted sympathetically.

"Perhaps Ellman left something in you after the first op and quietly extracted it at the second op," she said with a rueful smile.

"Don't be daft," I snapped. "I can do without that kind of black humour."

Without further comment Rita set up her Scrabble board on the bedside table and we were soon absorbed in a close-fought game.

I never sleep very well in hospital. Even in a separate room there is still a certain amount of noise. Nurses always seemed to be popping in to check my saline drip and catheter bag. That night I was also kept awake by the unpleasant smell of tobacco smoke drifting through the ward. Smoking in the hospital was only allowed in a few clearly defined areas, and was strictly banned in all wards. I suspected one of the nurses was having a quiet puff, perhaps in the day room or staff room. I was annoyed – it shouldn't be happening. It was a further example of the slip-shod standards which seemed to be pervading the hospital. Later the drip line became detached from the canula in my wrist. Fluid was dripping all over the sheets instead of into my vein. I rang my call bell for assistance. No-one came. I pressed the button again, listening this time for the distant sound of the buzz at the ward desk. I didn't hear anything, so I assumed the bell wasn't working. I resorted to shouting "nurse". It took about ten minutes to attract anyone's attention. I could have bled to death in that time. It just wasn't good enough. If I had been lying in bed at home with the phone beside me, I could have got an ambulance crew to my bedside quicker than I'd got help in this useless hospital. The nurse who eventually attended to me fixed the drip and then investigated why the bell hadn't worked. The lead was half out of the socket on the control panel, probably because no-one had bothered to check it despite the fact that I was a post-operative patient in a single room. It struck me I was paying a £35 a day amenity room charge just to have my health put in jeopardy.

During the Sunday, the drip and catheter were removed and I became a little more mobile, moving around my room and getting across the corridor to the loo. I was relieved to find I seemed to be recovering rapidly from the operation. Sunshine streamed into my room through the panoramic but rather dirty windows. It highlighted the thick layer of dust on the window sill. When had my room last been properly cleaned, I wondered? I got out of bed, took a paper towel from the dispenser above the basin, dampened it, and got to work, wiping down the window sill and my bedside table. This was preposterous, I reflected. Three days after an operation here I was cleaning my own hospital room. I threw the towel into the bin and carefully washed my hands. No way was I going to risk succumbing to MRSA. I wanted to go home. I'd be safer there and Mike would look after me better than the obviously disorganised nurses.

I spent the rest of the day brooding about falling NHS standards. Things had been much better in 1981. What was going wrong? Perhaps they'd let me go home tomorrow.

On the Monday morning I felt hungry for the first time since the operation. I was definitely on the mend and eagerly awaited the arrival of my bowl of cornflakes, my usual breakfast. It came in a covered plastic meal tray. I lifted the lid and then removed the cover over the plastic bowl. A steaming bowl of grey-coloured porridge confronted me. My stomach turned. I absolutely hate porridge. I burst into tears. Now they couldn't even get my breakfast order right. What could be simpler than bringing me a bowl of cornflakes? It was a relatively trivial incident, but for me it was the final straw. I was going home, right now. I pushed the breakfast tray aside and pulled out everything from my locker, stuffing it all into my bag. I dressed hurriedly and went to the day room to phone Mike for a lift. Then I sat on my bed beside my zipped-up bag and waited for him. He wouldn't be long as we only lived a mile from the hospital. I wrote a quick note to Mr Ellman, mentioning how dissatisfied I was with my care, that I was discharging myself for my comfort and well-being, and that I would be making a written complaint to the Chief Executive.

A nurse came in.

"I'm discharging myself," I said, seeing her surprised look.

"Why? What's wrong?"

"Just about everything."

She was a young nurse and looked anxious, almost scared.

"But it's nothing to do with you," I assured her. "The trouble comes from higher up."

"You'll need to sign a form. I'll get the doctor." Looking flustered, she disappeared.

I was signing the self-discharge form under the direction of a junior doctor when Mike appeared. He looked a bit dubious when he realised I was discharging myself, but soon accepted that I would be quite OK if I took it easy. He picked up my bag and we walked out to the car. Soon I was home again, so very relieved to be out of the mad-house that was Casterbridge General Hospital.

CHAPTER 4

Within a few minutes of arriving home I was sitting at my word processor, banging out a letter of complaint to the Chief Executive. There were five issues, as I thought I might as well include every incident indicative of poor standards. First the one I considered the most serious – why had an appointment for a pre-operative check been made for a date *after* the operation? Secondly, why had my call bell become detached from the control panel, a fault I regarded as potentially serious? Thirdly, why on one occasion had I not received my nightly heparin injection to prevent blood clots? I had been told supplies had run out –why? Fourthly, why was there a smell of tobacco smoke in the ward at night? And fifthly, just for good measure, why couldn't they even get a simple breakfast order right?

Mike posted it, and I felt I had got something off my chest. At last I was able to relax in the comfort and safety of my own home. My recovery was amazingly rapid. After a week or so I realised my bowel function was improving. After two weeks they were back to normal – no mucus, and decent-sized bits once or twice a day. In fact, I felt better than I had done from since the time of the first operation. Surely Ellman had done something. Perhaps something was wrong after the first op, and he had now put it right. I would ask him about it at my six-week check-up.

A few days after sending my letter to the Chief Executive, I had a phone call from the complaints department telling me to attend for the pre-operative urinary examination. I thought that was crazy, so I rang Dr Hick for advice. She rang back and told me the test was no longer necessary. She also told me that there were no cancer cells in the peritoneal fluid.

"I suppose that's good news," I remarked. "But it doesn't necessarily mean that there's no cancer in the mass, does it?"

She conceded that I was correct. She sounded very hesitant. The phone can often bring out characteristics in the voice which aren't always evident in face-to-face conversations. Once again I felt that she wanted to say something more.

While in hospital I had been told I was to have an MRI (magnetic resonance imaging) scan. This would tell the doctors more about the internal nature of the mass, and, presumably, would indicate the best treatment to use. I waited for the appointment to come. On the 3rd of October I had a phone call from some X-ray department asking why I hadn't shown up for the urinary test. I explained that I had been told it was not necessary. It seemed that Dr Hick hadn't thought to cancel the appointment, and I just assumed she had done. It was a lesson for me – never assume the NHS does anything. Be more hands on. Check everything yourself, then check it again. It might make me an extremely tedious patient but that was better than having the wrong leg chopped off, or whatever.

I eventually had a reply from the Chief Executive about my complaints. He conceded that they were justified and there followed the various assurances that procedures would be reviewed to ensure these things didn't happen again. It was all rather unconvincing whitewash, but there was nothing more I could do.

After a month of waiting I still hadn't got an appointment for the MRI scan. It had to be hands-on now. I phoned the MRI department as there was a possibility the appointment letter had been lost in the post. They appeared to have no knowledge of any request for the scan, but would investigate. Later I had a call from Mr Ellman's secretary.

"There is no need for an MRI scan at the present time," she enunciated carefully.

"But I was told I'd got to have one," I said.

"There is no need for an MRI scan at the present time," she repeated. It sounded like she was reading from a script from which she couldn't deviate.

I slammed down the phone. Why couldn't they have told me they didn't want a scan? Why keep me worrying about it? And why had they decided I didn't need a scan? How else could they investigate and monitor the mass? Then a thought struck me. I remembered Rita's jokey remark which I had instantly dismissed as the sick product of a mind addled by watching too many hospital soaps. Something had been left in me which was then surreptitiously removed. I wasn't having a scan because there was nothing to investigate. Suddenly everything started falling into place. If I took the 'foreign object' theory on board, it was almost like finding the missing piece from a jigsaw puzzle. Things started to make sense. I could see why so many confusing and odd things had happened. With the 'foreign object' scenario firmly in place, I went back to the beginning. Perhaps it was the explanation for all my post-operative pain and slow recovery, and later for the largely unexplained vaginal discharge and strange bowel problems. I guessed that Dr Foyle had been informed about the situation. No doubt he had been told that the plan was to open me up again on the pretext of finding a further mass. His partners would have been informed. Reassure her and try to treat any symptoms, but don't refer her back to the hospital, would have been their instructions, and they had followed them to the letter. 'Something mechanical' Dr Foyle had said. Had he been trying to drop a hint? No doubt he had qualms about what he was doing. Then there had been the very reassuring letter from Ellman about little chance of further disease. I suppose that was to try and stop me seeking treatment and investigations in the field of complementary medicine. But it hadn't stopped me. Terry Sutton's unconventional heat-seeking equipment had indeed shown something wrong in the pelvic area. Dr Hick's strange demeanour was now explained. She really had been trying to tell me something. She would have known exactly what had been going on, as she had assisted at the September operation. But she didn't dare to actually voice anything. Whistle-blowers don't advance in their careers, and Dr Hick was an ambitious young registrar looking for her first consultancy. I understood now why 'nothing' had been done at the operation. Anything removed had to go to the pathology lab. There would have been some raised eyebrows if non-human material was found. It also explained why no biopsy was performed – there was nothing suspicious from which to take a biopsy. Yes, everything fitted together perfectly. It was a Eureka moment.

I was soon due to see Ellman for my six-week check-up. I would confront him with my theory. It would be interesting to watch his reaction. But would I have the courage? I had the horrible feeling I would chicken out at the last minute and end up believing whatever cock and bull tale he would produce.

November the 6th found me in the waiting area of the outpatients' clinic. As usual, I waited and waited well past my appointment time. I mused that the term 'patient' must have been adopted because we have to be patient. Patience was a quality I sadly lacked, and these constant long waits made me anxious. I rehearsed in my head what I was going to say to Ellman. I wouldn't be too confrontational. I'd mention that my bowel problems had cleared up, suggesting he must have done something during the operation. Then I'd say something like, "I know it seems ridiculous, but it seems like you left something in me after the first op and removed it during the second one." 'Something' needn't necessarily be a foreign object – it could have been part of the cyst he had missed.

What would he say? He'd have to give me some kind of explanation.

At last I was called. I managed a strangled "hello" as I sat down at his desk. He was in his shirt sleeves and wearing red braces. I hate braces. Except for rotund men they are an unnecessary ostentation. With his heavy-rimmed glasses and rather aggressive pose, he reminded me of Larry King, the American TV anchorman. I was already on my guard.

"I got your note," he began. "Fancy complaining about the wrong breakfast."

This took me by surprise, as I hadn't mentioned my specific complaints in my note to him. Presumably the Chief Executive had sent him a copy of my formal complaints.

"I know that was trivial," I replied, "but I had other complaints as well."

"Maybe." He looked annoyed. "You don't know how lucky you are having an NHS."

I was flabbergasted. He made me feel like an ungrateful recipient of charity. Didn't he realise everyone paid for the NHS through their taxes? I'd paid my whack over the years and now it was pay-back time. And what were we doing wasting valuable consulting time entering into a discussion about the merits or otherwise of the NHS?

"Yes, we are lucky to have the NHS," I replied. "I've been in hospitals in the third world."

Suddenly he looked rather defensive. I felt quite pleased with myself by agreeing with him. I'd put him off his stride. Possibly my reference to third world hospitals suggested I had worked in the medical field. But his attitude infuriated me. There would be no holds barred now, no pussy-footing about.

"So what do you want to ask me?" he continued abruptly.

"I want to know about the nature of this lump and how you're going to treat it."

"You have this borderline cancer. We'll monitor you and perhaps give you a scan in about a year."

It didn't strike me as a sensible plan for someone on the verge of developing cancer and seemed to confirm that there wasn't really anything to monitor. Surely he wouldn't otherwise leave me for a year without some kind of scan.

"My bowels have been back to normal since the operation. That suggests you did something." I took a deep breath. "I think you left something in me after the first op and removed it at the second."

I watched him carefully. He seemed exasperated, but also extremely anxious. He looked down at my file and shuffled the papers, trying to straighten them.

"Now you listen to me. Let me explain things."

He was playing for time while he desperately tried to think up a feasible explanation for the rapid improvement in my bowel function.

"Your bowels are probably better because the mass was reactive swelling which has gone down."

"So you mean it went down naturally. It seems I've had an unnecessary operation. Couldn't you tell from the scan it was reactive swelling which would go down naturally?"

"No. Scans can't tell you everything. Because of the borderline cancer found in February, we couldn't take chances."

I was really confused now. In some ways I was glad that I had some kind of diagnosis. It was something I could latch on to and understand. It also seemed there was nothing much wrong with me at the moment. Not wanting to further antagonise someone who was about to stick his finger up my vagina, I kept quiet. He examined me and seemed satisfied.

"We'll have another CA125 blood test, and see you again in three months."

I was glad to get out. I charged out of the hospital, absolutely fuming. How dare Ellman speak to me as if I was a naughty schoolgirl? In fact, thinking back to the time when I was indeed a naughty schoolgirl, I think my teachers showed me more respect. What was the matter with the man? It was no way to treat a fifty-four year old woman. There had been no need for him even to raise the issue of my complaints as they were not against him personally, and had already been dealt with through other channels. I began to feel it was an attempt to throw up a smoke screen, an attempt to keep me away from considerably more serious issues. But Ellman was for it now. No one messes with me and gets away with it.

CHAPTER 5

Numerous friends had to endure my whinging and moaning about how the medics were treating me. I met with the polite sympathy I would have expected from them, but there was nothing any of them could do about it, and I think they all knew I was quite capable of dealing with matters myself. But there was one friend, Pam, at the Scrabble club, who, being a retired nurse, was more helpful than most.

"Ellman told me the mass was reactive swelling from the February op, which had gone down naturally," I explained to her one day after I'd duffed her up on the Scrabble board.

"Reactive swelling?" Pam looked confused.

"That's the phrase he used."

"But reactive swelling is something that goes down a week or two after an op. Well, that's what I've always understood it to mean."

"So it wouldn't persist for about eight months and then suddenly go," I replied.

"I wouldn't have thought so." She paused and looked me in the eye. "There's something odd going on."

"Do you think Ellman is trying to hide something?"

"Probably. I know the things these doctors get up to... you wouldn't believe... You've got to get your notes."

"What's the point? I wouldn't understand them."

"You would," Pam assured me. "You won't have peace of mind until you know what's been going on."

She was right. I was becoming obsessed with my 'foreign object' theory. Although it all seemed so perfect, it might not necessarily be correct. I remained very much aware that I had no medical training, and that even my knowledge of human biology was somewhat shaky. I pondered the term 'reactive swelling'. If I got a thorn in my finger, even a tiny one, I would develop considerable swelling around it because it would irritate the surrounding tissues. Once I had gritted my teeth and dug it out with a sterilised needle, the swelling would be gone within a day. So if something had indeed been left inside me, the swelling would have persisted until soon after the object had been removed. Now my theory attained even greater heights of perfection. It occurred to me that I had not asked Ellman a vital question – reactive to what?

I didn't obtain my notes as Pam had suggested. I had another appointment with Ellman in February 2001. I would give him one more chance to explain things properly to me. I would sit there until I fully understood everything. I would not allow myself to be brow-beaten into submissive acceptance.

At last the day of the next consultation arrived. Once more there was an interminable wait. I rehearsed my little speech in my mind – what was meant by 'reactive swelling'? What had my body been reacting to? Why had it gone away so quickly? They seemed reasonable questions. How would Ellman react? But would I even be seeing Ellman? I could be seen by 'a member of his team' as the appointment letter termed it. But then perhaps I'd get more out of the registrar, Dr Hick, or a junior doctor. I had to be prepared for anything.

About fifteen minutes after my 3.20 appointment time, Dr Hick came out of her consultation room carrying a file. That was a bit unusual, as the doctors usually got the nurses to do the running about. She strolled slowly through the waiting area, which was again unusual. Clinics always seemed to run late and the doctors and nurses always rushed around. She looked straight at me, and I looked back, meeting her eyes. Once more I got the feeling she was trying to tell me something. She entered the consulting room used by Ellman. A minute or so later she emerged without the file. Once more she caught my eye as she sauntered to the reception desk and handed the receptionist a bit of paper. This was totally unbelievable behaviour. I knew from previous experience that a patient is completely invisible to a doctor until it is their turn.

I had deliberately sat close to the reception desk so I could overhear what was going on. Soon after Dr Hick's antics, I heard one receptionist saying to another:

"No wonder Mr Ellman's running so late. He's seeing people he needn't see. Shouldn't he be doing diagnoses, not check-ups?"

That set me thinking. It seemed I might have been scheduled to see Dr Hick. She felt unable to deal with me, had told Ellman to add me to his list, had given him my file, and then informed reception of the switch. Ellman, no doubt, had added me to the end of his list. So, Dr Hick was standing her ground. She was no longer prepared to lie to me or kow-tow to Ellman. Perhaps she had another job lined up.

After waiting about forty minutes, I asked how much longer I would have to wait. I was told I was next on the list. Another fifteen minutes elapsed. Then someone else was called to Ellman's room, someone who had checked in far later than I had. It confirmed what I had suspected. Ellman had deliberately put me last on his list, no doubt in the hope that I would lose patience and leave. My rapidly increasing agitation was now compounded by raging anger. I wanted to go and smash Ellman's face in. Instead I got up and walked out. I had made up my mind. Ellman would now find himself the subject of an official complaint, and I would pursue him until he was struck off. He was devious and incompetent, his colleagues couldn't stand him, and there should be no place for him in the medical profession. If I didn't do something, no one else would. No doubt for years he had been protected by the fact that his largely middle-aged to elderly female patients had neither the time, the intelligence, nor the money to bring any kind of action against him, whereas I had ample amounts of all three. The rot had to stop.

Mike was supportive, although he could offer little help as to how I should pursue my complaint, as there were a number of avenues open to me. Friends were also unhelpful, although always sympathetic. No one I knew had ever made an official complaint, although nearly all had minor gripes about the NHS. The only specific advice I got was from Amy, another Scrabbler, who was a retired medical secretary.

"You'll be wasting your time," she warned me. "You'll never get anywhere. These doctors all stick together – I've seen it many times."

I ignored her. Amy had retired nearly twenty years ago. Things had changed since her time. Complaints procedures were better than they used to be, I reasoned. The public were generally more savvy about what went on, and were making more complaints, and bringing more successful legal actions. Yes, doctors had to be more accountable these days. I would succeed where others had failed. I was determined, and I would never give up.

My hairdresser, Viv, who had been regularly cutting my hair for nearly thirty years, was always a good listener, and seemed to quite look forward to the latest episode of my health woes. She was unusual in not having a TV, and I would joke that she didn't need the soaps because she had me. A good hairdresser with a regular clientele is a therapist as well. They hear it all, but it will never go beyond the privacy of the salon, which in Viv's case was a corner of her kitchen where she attended to clients on a strictly one-to-one basis. However, although confidentiality was never broken, Viv collated everything she heard. I have always maintained that if you want the low-down on the local gynaecologists you should ask a hairdresser. Sure enough, Viv came up trumps.

"You wouldn't believe what I've heard about Ellman. He is not liked."

'Not liked' was said with great emphasis, but beyond that her lips were sealed. But she seemed to think it was time someone had a go at Ellman. I began to feel that if I managed to get some kind of disciplinary action taken against him, it would benefit not only myself, but all the women of Casterbridge, and their long-suffering husbands and partners for that matter.

There were three avenues through which I could take action against Ellman. I could use the NHS complaints procedure, as I had with my earlier, relatively minor complaints. I could go to the General Medical Council, or I could find a solicitor who dealt with medical negligence and start a legal action. I immediately dismissed the third course. There simply wasn't enough evidence to prove my 'foreign object' theory. Besides, legal action cost money, which I had if need be, but would prefer not to spend. And another thing, I didn't want silly sums of compensation; I wanted truth and justice. Legal action would be a last resort.

I sought advice from the Community Health Council. They confirmed that I could use either the NHS complaints procedure or approach the GMC. They gave no advice on which course would be most appropriate, but I reasoned that as my complaint was very much about what I suspected was the unprofessional conduct of an individual doctor, the GMC was the place to go.

I wrote off to them with a full account of my experiences, which I thought built up to proof of my 'foreign object' scenario. No bloody sponge or swab could ever be produced, so it was inevitable that evidence would only ever be circumstantial. I also included a reference to Ellman's 'you're lucky to have an NHS' remark, which I felt wouldn't go down too well with the GMC as it indicated an arrogant and superior attitude totally out of keeping with the NHS ethical standards of the twenty-first century.

While I was working on my letter I received what could only be described as a grovelling written apology from Ellman about the delay in the out-patient clinic. He explained that it had been due to difficulty with an unusually slow senior house officer. He agreed that it was a totally unacceptable delay, and that he did not blame me at all for leaving. He was going to ask his secretary to arrange another appointment.

The letter made me highly suspicious. I would have expected a further appointment, possibly accompanied by an apology for the delay, from the clinic appointments staff. I did not, however, expect such a full apology from the consultant himself. Surely he had more important things to do. It was as if he wanted to get back on the right side of me, which seemed strange bearing in mind that I had accused him of leaving something in me. Surely he would be looking for an excuse to wipe his hands of me – get me passed to one of his colleagues, preferably in another hospital. But no. Ellman seemed rather desperate to hang on to me. Why? It occurred to me that if I consulted another gynaecologist, he or she would be confused by the sequence of events and might possibly say something that would incriminate Ellman. There would probably have to be some kind of letter of referral to a new consultant, and if indeed there was a cover-up going on, the new consultant would have to know about it. Although doctors are very prone to close ranks to protect each other, I wondered to what extent innocent colleagues would risk their livelihoods by allowing themselves to be drawn into a conspiracy. Some would play ball, no doubt, but some wouldn't. It seemed that Dr Hick had already decided to distance herself from the affair, and it was quite likely that other doctors would have the same attitude. It appeared quite obvious why Ellman wanted to hang on to me, but I was going to disappoint him.

My on-going care was low on my list of priorities. I felt completely well, and although I could understand that further check-ups and monitoring were desirable because of the very slight risk of cancer, I felt it was far more important that I probed for the truth about what had been going on. I didn't want the cover-up perpetuated under a new consultant. It would only take a few months to get things sorted, and the risk of anything developing in that period was minimal.

I decided to include the grovelling letter of apology in my submission to the GMC in the hope that they would regard it as suspiciously as I did. Finally everything was ready, and I posted quite a bulky letter.

I had a prompt reply acknowledging my complaint, enclosing a form to complete, asking for my medical records, and including details of the complaints procedure. It all seemed very efficient. I wrote to Casterbridge Hospital asking for my medical records from the year 2000. A few weeks later I received them. As far as I could tell, they were in order and nothing appeared to be missing. As Pam had said, I did understand most of them with the exception of pathology reports on blood tests which were just meaningless lists of figures. The hand-written notes on my consultations and operations appeared clear and accurate... Well, they corresponded with what I remembered I had been told. Just three items slightly surprised me. In October 2000 my case had obviously been discussed by oncologists in the cancer department and a letter had been sent to Ellman advising that monitoring of my condition was all that was necessary. Ellman had never told me he had referred my case to the cancer department, although I was relieved that he had done so. The second item was a pathology report on my 1981 cancer. I had not asked for any notes before 2000, but it seemed the 1981 pathology report had become mixed in with more recent notes, no doubt because it had been necessary to dig it out for reference. The third item was the last thing in the notes, about me walking out after the long wait at my February 2001 appointment. It said 'left with husband'. Mike had not been with me. Ellman had never emerged from his room, so could never have seen me and could not therefore have assumed that a man I may have been sitting next to was my husband. Only Dr Hick had met Mike. I guessed that what had happened was that Dr Hick had told Ellman I was waiting with my husband and that there could be trouble. Either she had made a genuine mistake about the identity of whoever was sitting next to me, or she had told him a deliberate lie to get herself out of seeing me.

I got all the notes photocopied and sent off to the GMC. Once that was done, I had time to study them in more detail. The histology report on my 1981 cancer intrigued me. Everything seemed correct – the dates, the description of the tumour (a papillary mucinous cystadenocarcinoma) and the name of the consultant pathologist, a Dr A Appleyard, but no signature. Yet there was something wrong about it. I studied it carefully. Of course! It was not the original report. The information appeared to have been obtained from elsewhere and typed on to current stationery. Casterbridge Hospital had not been an NHS Trust in 1981. The STD phone code had changed since 1981. The whole report therefore had a modern feel, and it could easily be mistaken for a report on tissues from either of the 2000 operations. In fact, that may almost have happened because I noticed a small mark under the '81', as if someone wanted attention drawn to it.

I knew that ancient medical notes were held on microfiche. No doubt doctors requiring copies could easily obtain them via the wonders of modern technology. Why then go to the trouble of typing the information on to new stationery? It was a fabricated report, and I felt it was designed to mislead. I wasted no time in writing to the GMC with my observations. It was further grist to the mill. I felt quite pleased with myself, quite the amateur sleuth in fact.

After the Harold Shipman case (the GP who murdered

hundreds of his patients) there had been much criticism of the GMC. To some extent it seemed to be a watchdog without bark or bite. I noticed from its letterhead that its motto was 'Protecting patients, guiding doctors'. From some of the things I had heard in the media 'Protecting doctors, ignoring patients' would seem more appropriate. But I had to be fair. From the information I had received it seemed that complaints were thoroughly investigated. Ellman would be given a month to respond to my allegations, and then I would have an opportunity to respond to his submission. The case would then go before a committee of doctors and lay people. The big problem with any kind of regulation of professionals is that it is only others in the same profession who are really in a position to judge their behaviour. Inevitably, there is a tendency to protect one's colleagues, and I believed that to be the case in the medical profession more than any other. I just hoped that the lay people had some clout, that they weren't token members of the committee to made things look fair and above board.

The complaint would take some months to process. I felt completely well. I reasoned that there was little point in seeking further care until the matter was sorted out. As things stood, a new consultant would be both wary and confused. Besides, I had no idea how I should go about finding a new consultant. Now that he knew about my complaint, Ellman would obviously refuse to deal with me. If he felt that regular checks on my condition were necessary, he would, no doubt, refer me to another gynaecologist, as it would be a breach of duty for him not to do so. If, on the other hand, my 'foreign object' theory was correct, check-ups would seem to be unnecessary, and might, indeed, reveal the subterfuge. A scan, for instance, might show that the lump shown on the previous scan had disappeared, which would be unlikely unless the 'reactive swelling' explanation was correct. I would just wait and see what happened, and if nothing happened, I would take it as further evidence that the 'foreign object' theory was correct.

Nothing happened, despite me being well overdue for a three-monthly check-up. Things were looking even better; my case was strengthening by the day. Working on the 'know your enemy' principle, I decided to find out more about Ellman. I went to the library and found his entry in the Medical Directory. There it was: James Johannes Ellman. He had qualified in 1972 in Pretoria, South Africa, but the very brief details in the entry indicated that he had soon left that troubled country for England. If he had been brought up in South Africa during the apartheid years, that might well explain the patronising and condescending attitude I had experienced. His middle name, Johannes, suggested he might have Afrikaans blood, perhaps being the offspring of a British-Afrikaans marriage. If so, he might have grown up under strong Afrikaaner influence, having it drummed into him that he was one of 'God's chosen people'. The concept of all people being equal would be alien to him, and he would have been taught that all races other than whites were inferior to him, and that even whites were a bit suspect unless they were of Boer stock. Despite his long time in England, perhaps his boyhood beliefs remained with him, but with racism being a no-no, his female patients were now the inferior group to be patronised and abused. I suddenly felt I had a much clearer understanding of Ellman.

The Medical Directory entry also gave his home address. I noted it, and a few days later took a slight detour to look at the Ellman abode. It was in Pine Grove, the very best part of town with the most expensive houses. His was an Edwardian-looking rambling pile nestling among dark and gloomy rhododendrons. They would look a picture for a few weeks in May and June, but would then be gloomy again. Although his house was well beyond my means, I didn't envy him. I'd never liked Pine Grove. It struck me as spooky with all the sombre pines and dark undergrowth. There were never any pedestrians because everyone went everywhere in their posh cars. It just didn't seem neighbourly. I couldn't imagine people chatting over their back fences while hanging out the washing.

As I hovered in the car near Ellman's drive, I wondered if he was mortgage-free, and how many little Ellmans there were to support. If he was struck off, which in my mind seemed increasingly likely, he would probably have to step a rung or two down the property ladder. Just so long as he didn't move into Heather Close, where Mike and I lived happily in our fairly modest detached house.

CHAPTER 6

After a month or so I received a copy of Ellman's response to the GMC regarding my complaint. I read it carefully. The general impression I got was that he had over-emphasised my trivial complaints, such as getting porridge for breakfast, to try and prove that I was a whinging, moaning, slightly paranoid housewife who could not be trusted. He also mentioned at some length the letter I had written to him before my first operation – the letter he claimed he had not received! This he termed 'slightly peculiar', again with the implication that I wasn't quite right in the head. All this didn't surprise me. It's fairly common knowledge that one of the principal defences of doctors is to try and prove that the patient is a bit mental.

It was much more difficult for me to judge issues relating to my clinical treatment. However, if a mass had remained in me after the September 2000 operation, I would have expected referral to a specialist centre where, possibly, a more skilled surgeon could have assessed the likelihood of a further successful operation, or another form of treatment. Doing nothing, as had happened, didn't seem a sensible option. It seemed surprising that there were no notes about the multi-disciplinary meeting in October 2000 where my case had been discussed. I began to wonder whether this meeting had actually taken place, especially as Ellman had never mentioned it to me.

I wrote back to the GMC with all my observations, adding the general conclusion that the nature of Ellman's response to my complaints had made me even more suspicious. Then there was another long wait. Ellman would have an opportunity to reply to my comments, and then the case would go before a screener who would decide whether there was cause for matters to be progressed further.

In early June I received a letter from the GMC stating that my care under Ellman had been satisfactory and that there were no grounds for a case of medical negligence or unprofessional conduct. However, doubts had been raised about aspects of my medical notes, but this was something the local heath authority should deal with rather than the GMC. I was extremely disappointed with their decision, and although there was no appeal procedure, I wrote asking if they might reconsider the case, especially in the light of what appeared to be irregularities in my medical records.

Someone calling themselves a senior case worker wrote back explaining that cases could not be reconsidered unless substantial new evidence was presented. She did, however, enclose details about making complaints under the Access to Heath Records Act of 1990.

So it all turned out as I feared it might. The GMC was indeed a watchdog without bark or bite, busy protecting heath workers except in the very rare cases where the unprofessional conduct was so blatant and open that it could not possibly be ignored. I had wasted an awful lot of time and effort. Yet I had been left with a glimmer of hope. There really were some doubtful aspects within my medical notes. I would have to follow them up. Perhaps somehow I would get Ellman through a weakness peripheral to the main case, a sort of attack on a flank.

I had, in fact, already started further investigations on my records. The fabricated histology report was extremely odd, although, perhaps, I was placing too much emphasis on this. Although it struck me as a rather clumsy attempt to mislead people about my condition, and had appeared to fail in this, there could be a perfectly reasonable explanation about why it had been done.

I began my investigation by phoning the medical records department. I made a general enquiry about the presentation of old medical records. Without giving my name I explained that I had found a twenty-year-old histology report retyped on up-to-date stationery. I was told quite clearly that this method was virtually unknown. It could possibly be done if original records were difficult to read, in which case a copy of the original record would be firmly attached to the new one. It was suggested that I checked whether or not this had been done. I did, of course, know full well there was no original report, but said I would have another look.

Then I wrote to the records department requesting a copy of the original 1981 histology report. I received a reply which mentioned a form I should complete which they had failed to enclose. I was intrigued to see that this letter had come from the medico legal section, not the records department. I phoned the number given to ask for the form to be sent, and was told it would be sent immediately. Two days later it had not arrived. I phoned again and was told there was no point in me pursuing the request because all my records prior to 1995 had been destroyed. This was apparently because I had gone for more than eight years without any contact with the hospital. It was explained to me that in such a case the records were destroyed at the beginning of the ninth year. The woman I was speaking to seemed to be in front of a computer terminal because I could hear tapping on a keyboard.

"Nothing before 1995," she said decisively. Why they couldn't have told me that at the time of my original request I don't know, but I was rapidly gaining the impression that nothing worked properly in the NHS.

I thought about the time scale of my infrequent visits to Casterbridge Hospital over the years. I had had my last check-up following the 1981 cancer in 1987. I had not visited the hospital again until July 1995 when I had a minor breast problem investigated. So I had missed this strange and what appeared arbitrary cut-off point by a few months. Presumably, if the breast problem had been investigated in 1994 my records would still be in existence. I would have thought that with a serious illness like cancer, which can reoccur at any time, all records would have been kept. I wasn't at all happy about the situation.

I turned my mind back to the fabricated document. If my 1981 records had been destroyed, how had Ellman found the information about my cancer which was printed on this document? The only other source would have been my GP's records, which are never destroyed. By the time they peg out, most patients have vast bundles. I suspected that a histology report from 1981 had found its way into my GP's notes. I phoned the receptionist at the surgery and asked about it, telling her I wanted it for some cancer research, which wasn't a lie – it was my research. Later she phoned back and said the cancer diagnosis was in the form of a letter from the hospital. She would not give me further details. I asked if I could have a copy, but she explained that because the document was pre 1990, and therefore not covered by the Access to Health Records Act, she would have to get permission from Dr Foyle.

I expected that was a mere formality, and was therefore very surprised when she phoned a day later and told me that Dr Foyle had not given permission for the release of the document. He had a right to do that, but why on earth should he? He had read the wording to me back in late 1999 when I had consulted him about the vaginal bleeding. It was hardly information that was unfamiliar and therefore possibly upsetting. The trouble was, I couldn't remember the exact words he had used, and I wanted to check that the wording and therefore the diagnosis had not been altered in some subtle way. So what did Dr Foyle know? Was he involved in this increasingly bizarre cover-up? Was he trying to protect Ellman? Or was he just being awkward for no particular reason?

I had never fully considered the possibility that Dr Foyle

knew exactly what had been going on, and was being directed by Ellman as to how to deal with me. But then I started thinking back. When I had gone to the doctor's about the vaginal discharge which had developed after the February 2000 operation, Dr Green, the partner I saw, said she would contact Ellman to ask about it. Two days later I popped into the surgery without an appointment just to ask if she had heard from him. By coincidence, she took a call from him while I sat in the waiting room. Her surgery door was open, so I could hear one side of the conversation. In fact, she said very little, but the call seemed very long, far longer than was necessary to tell her that the discharge was normal, which is what she later told me. Had Ellman been filling her in on the true situation – that there was something left in me which he intended to remove in September? Would ordinary GPs allow themselves to be drawn into such a cover-up? After all, they weren't exactly Ellman's close colleagues. Just how widely did the ranks close?

Then there had been Dr Foyle's odd remark a few months later – that my bowel problem was 'mechanical'. What had he meant? Why hadn't I asked him to elaborate? Was he trying to drop a hint? With the benefit of hindsight I would say that he was, but in early 2000 the 'foreign object' theory had not crossed my mind. I could not possibly have recognised then what he might have been implying.

So now I began to wonder whether I could trust my GPs. However, there was no point in launching into complaints against them. The evidence for collusion with Ellman was far too flimsy. I resolved to keep my eye on the ball – keep pursuing Ellman.

Because of the slight doubts voiced by the GMC about aspects of my health records, I decided to pin my hopes on the 'forgery' as I now termed the fabricated histology report. Forgery was a police matter. I prepared a brief summary of what I had found out so far, and took it, along with a bundle of my medical notes, to the Casterbridge Police Station. I talked at length to a sergeant in a private room, and he promised me that further investigations would be made. Now we were getting somewhere. Ellman was a criminal. He could even be banged up. Struck off and banged up – just what he deserved!

My fantasies came to an abrupt end a few days later when the police phoned me to explain that they didn't think it was a police matter. I just couldn't believe it. Since when was forgery not a police matter?

It was now nearly the end of July 2001. Almost six months had passed since I had decided to pursue Ellman, but I had got nowhere. However, there remained one more course of action – the NHS complaints procedure. Perhaps that would bring results. It was a complicated three-stage process, probably deliberately made as daunting as possible to put off all but the most determined complainants. Firstly there would be an internal investigation. If that wasn't satisfactory, I could request an independent review, and finally the case could go to the Health Ombudsman. I could envisage it taking months, so it was fortunate that I remained in good health. After my experience with the GMC I was also concerned about how open and honest such an investigation would be. Wouldn't it just be another case of doctors banding together to protect one another? Just how could you find a chink in the closed ranks?

Despite my doubts, I went ahead, at first writing to the Chief Executive of Casterbridge Hospital. I informed him of both the GMC investigation, and my contact with the police. I wanted him to be fully aware of how seriously I regarded the matter. I then listed a number of specific questions to which I required answers. These were carefully formulated and reference made to sections of my medical notes where necessary.

My first question was about the fabricated histology report.

I demanded to know why the document had been drawn up in such a way, how and when information was obtained, who formulated the document, and was the information accurate.

My next question was did I still have my cervix? I had noticed that on a pathology lab report that my cervix had been listed as going to the lab, but that they had not received it. So was my cervix still in me, or had it been lost in some dusty corridor, and possibly eaten by rats? Or had Ellman retained it and had it on toast for breakfast. (I did not, of course, include these fantasies in my letter.)

Thirdly I questioned the reasons for the sudden onset of a vaginal discharge a month after my February operation. Ellman had told the GP that it was normal, but from the hospital notes it appeared they suspected an infection.

Next I asked about the terminology used for a cancer which occurs nineteen years after a previous one. Was it 'recurrent' or 'new'? I also questioned whether the oncologists studying my case had been confused by the fabricated histology report. I remembered that Ellman had admitted to the GMC that there had been some uncertainty during the multi-disciplinary meeting.

Other questions concerned my bowel problems. I asked what might have caused them, and why the problems immediately cleared up after the second operation. I had noticed that Ellman had written in my notes during the November 2000 consultation that my bowels were a problem, when I had told him the problems had cleared up. I suggested that he had written this lie to support the suggestion that the lump was still inside me.

I asked why a biopsy had not been taken during the September 2000 operation, pointing out that this seemed to be a vital procedure in someone with suspected cancer.

I pointed out that no letter detailing the September 2000 operation had been sent to my GP, as was normally the case. I asked why it had not been sent, and even suggested it might have been removed from my file before photocopying because of the information it contained. Once more I found myself wondering how deeply Dr Foyle was involved in the cover-up.

Next I asked why I had not been given the MRI scan I had been promised after the September 2000 operation. Surely, if a lump remained in me some kind of scan was very important.

I asked for a copy of the results of the CA125 blood test I had had in November 2000. It had surprised me that this information had not been given to me, but I supposed it had been because I had not attended follow-up appointments. No doubt I would have heard something if it had been raised. I assumed that no news was good news.

Finally, I raised issues about my amenity room for the September 2000 operation. I pointed out that it was surprising that one was available seeing I was admitted at ten days' notice. I also mentioned that when I told the house officer who did my pre-op checks that I was happy to pay for peace and quiet, he said the room was 'on the NHS' despite the fact that I had signed an agreement to pay. However, I never received the bill for £140 to cover my four-day stay.

I thought about that point for a while. In February 2000 I had also asked for an amenity room, but at the time of admission none was available. Miraculously, one became available the morning after my operation. I spent the rest of my stay in it and was properly billed. Why had it suddenly become available? In general, Casterbridge folk weren't poor, and older patients especially were happy to pay for privacy and peace while receiving NHS care. The few amenity rooms, which were simply side rooms off the main ward, were usually over-subscribed. On many occasions they were used by non-paying patients where there was a need, such as when infection control was necessary. So why on earth was I thought worthy of having an amenity room in February and again in September, when I wasn't even charged for it? My fertile imagination went into overdrive. Of course! After Ellam had realised his mistake during the February operation, there was, no doubt, a possibility that I would have had another operation if the foreign object caused severe problems. Wheeling a patient back to the operating theatre in front of a lot of anxious on-lookers who had probably overheard snippits of conversation among the medical staff, didn't exactly inspire confidence. Then there was the 'unsuccessful' outcome of the September operation. Ellman knew that patients talk among themselves, passing around their opinions and concerns about the medical staff, but that those in separate rooms have far less contact with fellow patients. If something dodgy was going on, keeping the patient isolated was probably a priority. I strongly suspected that the amenity room I had had in September had been booked months previously, and that there had been no intention of billing me for it.

Having worked out what seemed a satisfactory scenario, I brought my mind back to the task in hand. My long letter of complaint was posted off to the Chief Executive along with my medical notes, carefully numbered to indicate the matters on which I had queries.

I knew that I would have to wait about a month for a reply, but given the complexity of my complaints, and the fact that we were now into the summer holiday period, I expected to have to wait even longer. I also expected that my complaints would not be satisfactorily addressed, and that I would probably end up going to the Health Ombudsman.

CHAPTER 7

My complaint to the Chief Executive had been posted on the 31st of July 2001. The full reply was dated 3 September, although, to be fair, I had received a letter before that to warn me that enquiries were taking longer than anticipated. That didn't surprise me at all. I could envisage numerous frantic meetings between the Chief Executive, Ellman, and other medics, to mix some kind of whitewash which might just provide a thick enough cover-up. Some hopes I thought, as I unfolded the bulky letter.

The first point dealt with was the fabricated histology report. It was explained that records from the 1980s had been placed on microfiche and that it was easier to reproduce them on to new stationery than to photocopy from the microfiche. By way of back-up, enclosed was what was described as the original request form from 1981, along with the pathologist's hand-written comments. I glanced at them briefly. The so-called request form appeared merely to be a form showing my admission with suspected appendicitis. The pathologist's comments, which were the exact words typed on to the new stationery, were simply written on a plain piece of paper. Why on earth could they not have sent a copy of the actual form held on microfiche?

I had not got beyond the first page of the letter, and already I was suspecting major shenanigans. I knew nothing about the problems of reproduction from microfiche, but I thought it reasonable to suppose that a modern system designed to hold something as important as medical records would be able to reproduce a copy at the touch of a button. It appeared that the form relating to my admission had been reproduced in this way as it was hand-written on pre-printed stationery. So why hadn't the pathology report been reproduced in the same way? Something very odd was going on. Then there was the fact that I had already been told my pre-1995 records had been destroyed. Transferral to microfiche was hardly destruction. I had been lied to. Why?

I moved on to the next paragraph which concerned the removal or otherwise of my cervix. It seemed the Chief Executive was waiting for further clarification from Ellman, and would write again.

My question about the unusual vaginal discharge was answered by Ellman's suggestion that it was old blood from the sub-total hysterectomy. It couldn't have been, as the discharge was watery, not bloody. Perhaps I should have been more accurate with my information, but surely it was up to the medics to ask the questions where doubt could exist?

Although the radiologist's methods of operation were detailed, my question about when cancer was termed 'new' or 'recurrent' was not answered. There seemed to be a general policy to obscure and confuse issues with irrelevant details. It was something politicians did when being intensely questioned by interviewers like Jeremy Paxman. Sometimes even he couldn't cut through the waffle. What hope was there for me?

Apparently Ellman could not explain why my bowel function had suddenly improved. Further enquiries were to be addressed to the bowel specialist who performed the sigmoidoscopy before the September operation. Ellman's explanation for why he had not taken a biopsy of the lump was that an attempt had caused bleeding. So what, I thought. I was in a modern operating theatre with methods for stopping bleeding, and transfusions immediately available. Little risk would have been involved, and much information about the lump would have been obtained. It struck me as very poor judgement.

The fact that no report on the operation had been sent to my GP was explained as an administrative oversight. I continued to think otherwise. Either it had been removed from my file because it contained sensitive information, or there had never been any intention to write one in the first place. So many things could be easily explained by 'administrative oversights'.

As regards my question about why I did not have the MRI scan which had been requested, it was explained that the multidisciplinary team who discussed my case thought that occasional ultrasound scans would be adequate for monitoring my condition. I felt unable to dispute this, although it had been a pity they had not told me of their decision.

The next point dealt with issues raised at the fraught November consultation. Ellman claimed he had written 'bowels a problem' because I had told him that. It was a blatant lie. I had told him my bowel problems had cleared up. I suspected it was not a case of him not listening properly, but more a case of him manipulating things to suit his own ends. He also denied to the Chief Executive that he had used the term 'reactive swelling'. Another lie. It was a phrase I instantly latched on to as a possible explanation as to why my bowel function had improved. It wasn't the sort of thing I could have dreamt up.

A copy of my November 2000 CA125 test was enclosed. It was 30, which was lower than it had been in January and August (95 and 35 respectively). That seemed good, but I had no way of knowing what was regarded as a normal reading.

Finally it was explained that I had not been billed for my amenity room because I had been so dissatisfied with the standard of care I had received. That seemed ridiculous – it suggested that anyone in an amenity room could have their bill waived if they complained about anything. I stuck to my original belief that the room had been booked for me, and that there had never been any intention of charging me. Once more I recalled the brief conversation I had had with a junior doctor when I attended for my pre-op checks in September 2000.

"I hope I get an amenity room," I had said. "I don't mind paying for peace and quiet."

"But it's on the NHS," he replied.

I thought he was just a bit wet behind the ears. "Yes, I know the treatment is on the NHS," I said, "but if I want an amenity room I have to pay for it, don't I?"

He didn't say anything, and the matter wasn't raised again. Surely even a junior doctor would have known about the amenity room system. It really did suggest that my admission to a side room had been pre-planned.

To conclude, the letter had not provided sensible answers to any of my queries. In fact, some of the explanations were so preposterous that I had become even more suspicious about what had been going on.

"It's a massive cover-up," I screamed at Mike, as I threw the letter down in front of him. I knew he was taking a far more calm and detached view of the matter. Perhaps he would detect things I hadn't noticed, or had refused to accept. His analytical accountant's mind would weigh things up, sort the wheat from the chaff, and perhaps come up with a rather different view of things. Perhaps I was just getting too emotional about the whole thing. He spent about ten minutes reading carefully through the letter.

"It's very unsatisfactory," he concluded calmly. "If anything, it raises more questions than it answers. I suppose now you'll have to go on to the next stage."

"Of course I will," I replied, relieved that Mike was in total agreement with me.

The next stage in the NHS complaints procedure was the Independent Review. My complaint would be considered by an especially trained person called a Convenor assisted by an independent lay person. Even before I commenced on this stage, I had my doubts about the true independence of the independent lay person. I had become really cynical. I suspected that this review would do little more than rubber-stamp the findings of the internal enquiry. It might raise some minor criticisms just to try and convince me that it had done the job properly, but basically it would be in general agreement with the findings of the Chief Executive.

Off went another long letter to the Chief Executive. I made clear my dissatisfaction with his explanations and asked for the complaints to be considered for an Independent Review. I then made some lengthy comments about some of his findings and explanations.

I pointed out that the medical records department had previously told me that my pre- 1995 records had been destroyed. Therefore I could conclude that the photocopies of microfiched records I had been sent were either fakes, or that the medical records staff were so poorly trained that they did not understand the system. I also pointed out that the photocopy did not include the name of Dr A Appleyard, suggesting there may be other records from which this information was obtained. I made clear that I still regarded the 1981 histology report as fabricated, and designed to mislead.

I pointed out that the vaginal discharge I had suffered had been watery, not bloody. I suggested that it had been prevented from draining out after the operation due to blockage by the foreign object. The object had then shifted, allowing the fluid to escape, but putting pressure on the bowel instead.

I asked that the bowel consultant should be made aware of the quite sudden onset of my bowel problems about a month after the first operation, and of how quickly they cleared up after the second.

I suggested that Ellman and Dr Foyle, my GP, had colluded to conceal from me what had happened during the February 2000 operation. This could explain why, despite my persistent bowel problems, Dr Foyle had not referred me back to the hospital, instead deciding to wait for the routine scan to 'discover' the lump. I also suggested that Ellman did not entirely trust Dr Foyle, which was why, during the November 2000 consultation, he had asked me to contact him direct if I had any problems.

For a moment I stopped my frantic pounding of the keyboard of my ageing word processor. It was awful to think that my own GP, someone who had known me and occasionally treated me for nearly eighteen years, could possibly think that protecting a colleague was more important than doing the best for his patient. How on earth could he allow himself to be drawn into the conspiracy? Wasn't he putting his own career in jeopardy? I could just about understand doctors not telling tales about each other, but I could not understand how someone could risk their own career to protect a colleague. It seemed to me that strange forces were at work. It was like some secret brotherhood with terrible oaths and rituals. It was evil and frightening.

I pulled myself together. This ridiculous fantasising would get me nowhere. Anyway, I told myself, the medical profession was more open these days. People did whistle-blow. That was how the unsatisfactory baby heart operations in Bristol had been revealed, and it had been a fellow GP who had raised queries about the high death rate among Shipman's patients. Yes, there were decent doctors out there, but perhaps they were a bit thin on the ground. They all had their own careers to think about, and could not risk being professionally ostracised. All my doubts came flooding back.

I returned to the letter. I asked why there was no clear diagnosis of the lump, pointing out that in a letter to Dr Foyle,

Ellman referred to it as a 'presumed cyst'. I pointed out that it did seem strange that no one had used any clear medical terminology to describe the lump.

Finally I made a snide comment about the decision not to charge me for the amenity room, suggesting that so long as a patient complains enough, the payment will be waived.

The letter went off on the 18th of September 2001, and I settled down for another long wait. How much longer would it be before I got things sorted? If this stage was unsuccessful, the next stage was the Health Ombudsman, but perhaps that wouldn't be necessary.

While the Convenor was conducting his so-called Independent Review, the Chief Executive wrote to assure me that I did have my cervix because I had had a sub-total hysterectomy. There was no explanation as to why the cervix had been listed as going to the pathology lab when it was still in me. It suggested sloppy practices in the operating theatre, and it could also have been sloppy practice that had caused a swab or sponge to have been left in me. These things are meant to be carefully counted before a patient is sown up. One way and another, it seemed people did not have their minds on the job on the 1st of February 2000. Was it because they were all rabbiting on about the Shipman sentence which had been announced the previous afternoon, and had dominated the media all evening? It must have been a major, and disturbing, topic of conversation.

The Independent Review should have been completed within a month, but at the end of October the Chief Executive wrote again to inform me that it would take a few more weeks. This did not surprise me, given the extensive and complicated nature of my complaints. It was better to have the inquiry conducted properly than to insist on adherence to an unrealistic timetable. His letter also contained an explanation from the bowel consultant about why my bowel problems had cleared up after the second operation. He suggested that part of the mass could have been a haematoma (a sort of blood blister) which collapsed when Ellman attempted a biopsy. This would explain the bleeding he reported. To some extent this explanation sounded feasible, but I found it difficult to believe. Surely any surgeon would recognise a haematoma, and I would have been told at the time that it was the probable cause of my problems, and that it had been drained. I became even more suspicious. Surely, surely this Independent Review would get to the bottom of things.

CHAPTER 8

After nine weeks the Independent Review had still not been completed. This was now about twice the recommended time scale, and my patience was beginning to run out. I kept telling myself that it was because the Convenor was being thorough, and would therefore root out the truth. On the other hand, it would also take time to mix and apply a really impenetrable coating of whitewash. I wrote once more to the Chief Executive, complaining about the delay, and also commenting on the bowel consultant's suggestions. I implied that there may have been some collusion between him and Ellman. I also said I was becoming increasingly suspicious, and that if they thought delaying tactics would make me go away, they could think again. I threatened to go on hounding them until I got to the truth.

I finally received the report from the Convenor at the end of November. This Convenor turned out to be a retired Air Vice Marshall. What were his qualifications for conducting such an inquiry? He sounded too 'establishment' for my liking. I could imagine the sort of things being said within the upper echelons of the NHS when he was appointed – 'decent chap, safe pair of hands, won't rock the boat, one of us'. In other words he was a respected pillar of society, like doctors. It was all the old boys' network. So what hope was there that I, Monica Bland, a nobody housewife, could break through the closed ranks?

To give him his due, the Air Vice Marshall had indeed been very thorough. The letter ran to twelve pages including the report from the Independent Clinical Advisor he had appointed. It appeared that every point I had raised had been considered. However, even before I started reading through it, I suspected that the powers that be were well aware by now of my intelligence and tenacity and that a super-opaque coating of whitewash had therefore been thickly brushed on. Issues would be buried under masses of technical medical details that I would barely understand. It would give the impression of a thorough inquiry, when, in fact, it was largely designed to confuse and obscure. I felt I was beginning to get the hang of things as I started to read the report with more than my usual degree of scepticism.

The report began with an apology for the delay in processing the case, the explanation being that it had been necessary to arrange a face-to-face meeting with the Independent Clinical Advisor (a consultant gynaecologist from a centre of excellence some distance away).

My suggestion that the 1981 histology report was fabricated was dismissed. The Convenor made it clear that proper procedures had been followed. The report continued in similar vein – dealing with each point I had raised and concluding that the internal enquiry had dealt with it fairly, and that the explanations I had received for confusing events were reasonable. Where medical details and procedures were involved, the input from the Clinical Advisor was included. There was no attempt to obscure the facts under unnecessary waffle, and in that respect I had to concede that the Convenor had produced a clear and easily understandable report. However, all he had really done was rubber-stamp anything that the Chief Executive had already said. There was no criticism of medical decisions or procedures. Where my memory of what was said at consultations with Ellman differed from what he had written in my notes, the matter was dismissed because of lack of evidence. In other words, where there was a clear difference of opinion, such as when I told Ellman my bowels were no longer a problem, and he wrote down 'bowels a problem' it was the consultant who was to be believed. If only I had secretly recorded that consultation! That really would have been damning for Ellman.

The Convenor concluded that it was not necessary to appoint an independent panel to review my complaints as in his opinion they had already been satisfactorily dealt with during the internal enquiry. He went on to point out that I could take my complaints to the Health Ombudsman if I was dissatisfied with his decision.

Needless to say, I was extremely dissatisfied with his decision. I wrote him a reasonably polite letter thanking him for the time and effort he had devoted to my case, and informing him that I was now taking the matter to the Ombudsman. At this point I decided to make him aware of another matter I had been investigating while he was preparing his report. It could, possibly, make him change his mind about whether to set up an independent review panel.

The subject of my personal investigation had been the hand-written histology request form and subsequent report dating from 1981. It was my belief that these documents were not genuine copies from the original microfiched records. Even during my initial brief perusal of them, I had the feeling there was something not quite right about them. At a later date I studied them much more closely.

The histology request form did appear to be a genuine 1981 style layout. My name and address, NHS number, date of birth, and GP at the time were all typewritten and correct. They would have been attached to the original form on a sticky label – one from a number pre-prepared and kept in my file. There was also a large laboratory number which had the appearance of being generated by a hand-held stamping machine. The various sections of the form were filled in by what appeared to be two, or possibly three, different forms of handwriting. Details of the consultant, the ward, and the date, were filled in with a firm, upright hand. Details of the specimen, the clinical details, and diagnosis were filled in with a forward-sloping loopy-style writing, the writing used to describe the specimen (rt ovarian tumour) being slightly more loopy and old-fashioned-looking than the rest, but not so different that it could not have been written by the same person.

I recognised the writing. It was Ellman's, I was sure it was. I found my bundle of medical notes and flipped to a page covered with his scrawled consultation notes. I placed the histology request beside it. It was the same writing. The forward slope was the same, the letter formation was the same. Or was I imagining things? Could Ellman have forged the document, possibly with the help of other members of his team? I thought about how he could have done it. Perhaps he had found a 1981-style request form in another patient's file. He could have scanned it into a computer, scrubbed out the original details, and just printed out the form itself. Then he could have filled in my details.

I was intrigued to see that in the 'specimen' box 'appendix' had been written in the upright hand and then crossed out. Had the form been partly filled in before the operation had commenced back in 1981? I very much doubted whether such a thing would ever be done, and even if it was, I imagine the form would have been thrown away and a new one made out to avoid any possible confusion. It was as if the crossing-out had been deliberately put on this fake form in an attempt to add authenticity. But why go to all this trouble? I began to get the feeling that the Chief Executive had been greatly concerned about the fabricated 1981 histology report and had questioned Ellman closely about it. Ellman had therefore been forced into producing back-up evidence even though this too appeared to be fabricated. He was digging himself in deeper and deeper. Did the Chief Executive realise what Ellman was doing? Surely he must have noticed the similarity in the handwriting. Was he just turning a blind eye, or was he actively involved?

With all these questions churning around in my head, I turned to the histology report itself, which was two different pieces of handwriting on plain paper. Perhaps Ellman had been unable to locate a genuine 1981-style histology report form, I speculated with growing cynicism. The first paragraph described the specimen, while the second paragraph dealt with the diagnosis (a papillary mucinous cystadenocarcinoma of the ovary). Once again, the writing in the second paragraph looked familiar, although I could not immediately place it. I went back to my medical notes, studying the variety of handwriting. As well as Ellman's loopy scrawl, there were short comments written and forms filled in by numerous doctors on his team. A pre-admission check form filled in by a Dr Kemp caught my eye. The small, upright writing looked exactly the same as that on the histology report, and also the same as some of the writing on the request form. My eye was drawn particularly to a figure '8' which happened to appear on both forms. It had been written in a way whereby the join was at the left hand of the top circle rather than the much more common right. I even got out my magnifying glass to check more carefully. It was a very unusual way to write an '8'.

So it seemed Ellman had dragged his junior staff into the ever-increasing mess. Perhaps they had not realised exactly what they were doing. But perhaps they did. It was Dr Kemp who had let slip that my amenity room was to be 'on the NHS'. Had that been a genuine slip-up, or had he been trying to convey something to me in an indirect way, as had Dr Hick with her strange eye-contact? I felt genuinely sorry for these young doctors. They would be relying on good reports from Ellman to progress in their careers. Whistle-blowing, or even a reluctance to co-operate in anything underhand could jeopardise their futures. What were they to do? What would I do in that situation?

I sat at my desk, my head in my hands, not knowing what to think or what to do. Everything seemed so confusing. Why had a fabricated histology report been produced in the first place? I was quite sure it would have been much easier to have reproduced the original report from the microfiche. The only explanation did indeed seem to be that it had been designed to confuse Ellman's oncology colleagues into thinking I had active cancer in 2000 and therefore giving me chemotherapy, as had vaguely been promised after the September 2000 operation. The trouble was, the ruse had been discovered. Even though the histology report looked contemporary, some sharp-eyed individual had noticed it related to 1981 and had underlined the date to draw attention to it. And that is why I did not, fortunately, get chemotherapy I did not need.

For a moment I had the feeling that the disorientating fog around the whole affair was beginning to lift and that I could see things more clearly. Then it would all descend again as I considered other aspects of the case. Was I missing something quite obvious? It was so easy to get into a pattern of thinking which might be based on entirely incorrect assumptions. Another problem was that I kept going off at tangents. I returned to the handwritten documents. Perhaps the writing was by different people. Most older people of Ellman's generation have forward-sloping loopy writing. It was how they were taught in primary school in the forties and fifties. Most younger people have upright styles closer to italic because that was how they were taught, and many form their letters and numbers in odd ways because they were not taught properly. I would ask Mike and a few friends if the writing specimens looked the same to them, and then I would consult a handwriting expert.

Mike immediately noticed a similarity. So did all my friends.

The general comment was, 'I'm no expert but....' I found a local handwriting analyst in the Yellow Pages and phoned him to check his credentials and explain what I wanted him to do. I feared he might be one of those people who just did character assessments from handwriting, but it turned out that he was trained in forensic work, regularly worked on cases of forgery, and was used to giving evidence in court. I'd hit on just the right person. His fees seemed sensible. He reckoned that what I wanted him to do would cost about £50, a sum I could easily afford.

I sent off clear photocopies of all the necessary documents. About a week later I received the report. The analyst was quite sure that Ellman had written the clinical details and diagnosis on the histology request form. He quoted as evidence the degree of slope of the writing, the style, and the formation of particular letters. He was only eighty per cent certain that one of the paragraphs on the histology report had been written by Dr Kemp. He explained that this was because he had very limited material with which to work, as the pre-admission check form only included a few words and numbers. But eighty per cent was good enough for me.

So it appeared the histology report was fabricated, the information, no doubt, having been cobbled together from various sources, my GP's notes probably being the main one. The back-up documentation was forged. Surely this was a criminal offence. I looked once more at the fabricated histology report. The consultant pathologist who had produced it was a Dr A Appleyard. This name did not appear on the back-up documentation. So from where had Ellman obtained this name? Perhaps it was contained within my GP's notes, or perhaps he had simply asked around about who had been in that post in 1981. No doubt some long-serving member of staff would have known. It really did seem Ellman had gone to great trouble to produce an authentic-looking fabrication.

I wrote to the Health Ombudsman on the 13th of December 2001. I gave him the background to my complaints – that they had been rejected by the GMC, that the internal NHS inquiry had been unsatisfactory, and that the Convenor had not granted an Independent Review. I tried to simplify my complaint as much as possible. I explained that I thought absorbent material had been left in me after the February 2000 operation, and that it had been surreptitiously removed in the September 2000 operation. I accepted that there could be two other possible scenarios: the lump could have grown rapidly between the two operations. I calculated that from the microscopic beginnings in February, which might have been missed during the operation, the lump would have needed to double in size every ten days to have reached the size shown in the 24th of August ultra-sound scan. Assuming it would have gone on growing between then and the 21 of September operation, it would have been enormous. But this had not happened. I concluded that the lump had not been growing at all, or only extremely slowly. That would lead to the second scenario – that Ellman had missed quite a substantial and possibly cancerous mass during the February operation. That would clearly be a case of medical negligence. But given that nothing was done to treat this apparently inoperable mass, the 'foreign object' scenario seemed the most likely.

I went on to mention what I believed was the role played by all the doctors associated with my case, and suggested that there was a widespread conspiracy to cover up what had actually happened.

I also enclosed details of my investigations into the various suspicious handwritten documents. It was my increasingly strong opinion that my findings in this area would arouse concerns and that this would trigger a full investigation.

I toyed with the idea of including evidence from Terry Sutton, my complementary therapist. He had carried out thermal imaging of my pelvic area in June 2000 and again in

June 2001. The June 2000 images had shown a hot area around the uterus, suggesting inflammation or even cancer, but this had disappeared in June 2001. In June 2001 a Russian expert in thermal imaging, who was working with Terry to train complementary practitioners how to use this diagnostic tool, looked at the two images. Terry had made sure she had no prior knowledge of my case except that I had had two operations – in February and September 2000. She spoke little English, so we had to use an interpreter. In translation it came out that she thought 'packing' was the cause of the hot-spot seen in June 2000. That really did support my own suspicions, which were shared by Terry. Perhaps this Russian doctor, who had used thermal imaging techniques for many years, had come across similar situations before. No doubt practices in Russian operating theatres were even sloppier than our own.

I looked closely at the coloured computer printouts generated by the thermal imaging equipment. They would not mean much to any medic unfamiliar with the technique, which was just about everyone within conventional medicine. Terry himself had suggested that the hot area could be due to post-operative scar tissue. It all seemed too complicated and inconclusive, so I decided in the end not to include it.

The letter, along with all the bulky enclosures, went off to the Health Ombudsman. It was my last chance, the final stage of the NHS complaints procedure. I was reasonably confident that this time I would get results. The evidence surrounding the fabricated and forged documents seemed pretty damning. But with Christmas intervening I knew I would have to wait until well into January for the Ombudsman's decision.

After Christmas Mike and I flew to Cape Town from where we took a cruise to the far-flung island of St Helena. I wanted to get away from it all. But however far you go, however remote the destination, your body and your thoughts are always with you. What had been going on in my pelvis? What could still be going on? I wouldn't rest until I knew.

CHAPTER 9

My holiday caused the Ombudsman to delay his investigation into my case. Despite the fact that I had sent him my medical notes, he required a further set direct from Casterbridge Hospital, for which my permission had to be obtained. I dealt with the necessary paperwork directly I returned home on the 19th of January. However, I still had to wait until late March for the Ombudsman's decision on whether or not to investigate my case.

The letter from the Investigation Officer ran to three pages, but my hopes were shattered by the first paragraph. It had been decided not to investigate my complaint. The decision had been reached in consultation with a consultant gynaecologist – just another example of doctors protecting each other, I thought with my usual cynicism. The rest of the letter explained why they had not taken matters further.

It was recognised that my principal complaint was that absorbent material had been left inside me after the February 2000 operation. Suddenly, in the same paragraph, 'absorbent' was changed to 'absorbable'. In other words, material such as a swab or a sponge, or 'packing' as the Russian interpreter had termed it, had become material which was designed to be absorbed and destroyed gradually by the body, like material used for stitching. They were two quite different things, and if the Ombudsman thought I could believe otherwise, he must have been under the impression that I had just fallen off the top of the Christmas tree. With increasing anger I read on.

There was no explanation as to why I had not received any further treatment for the inoperable mass. The improvement in my bowel function was explained by the fact that the bowels would have been moved about during the September 2000 operation, which suggested to me that the bowels had not been put back correctly after the February operation. There was no concern about the fabricated and forged medical records because they said pathology records were kept separately from patients' medical notes, and were not destroyed. Nothing was said about why the report did not appear on a proper form, or how the name Dr A Appleyard had been obtained. It was my immediate view that in this area their investigations had not been at all thorough. The only point on which there was slight criticism was that I had not been informed of the CA125 test result as soon as possible after it was done. It was pointed out that this was not a particularly serious issue, and I had to agree, bearing in mind that I had not attended the appointment at which I would have been told the result.

I showed the letter to Mike and he agreed with me that it was a total whitewash. In fact, of the three stages the complaint had now gone through, this last stage was definitely the most superficial and disappointing. We both felt that the Ombudsman's role was simply to rubber-stamp the previous enquiries. I was rapidly reaching the conclusion that the NHS complaints procedure was a complete sham, deliberately designed to discourage patients from pursuing complaints, and only accepting liability in the most blatant and easily provable cases of malpractice. It would be a complete waste of time to ask the Ombudsman to reconsider some of the issues. It would only result in yet another coat of whitewash. I would now have to consider other avenues. I was not going to give up.

What options were left? There was legal action, obviously. But I was reluctant to follow that course. It would be very expensive, and I was not after massive compensation because, as far as I knew, I was now in good health. I just wanted to know what had been going on. If there were inaccuracies in my medical records, I wanted them corrected, and if there had been malpractice and cover-ups, I wanted those responsible to be disciplined appropriately. The ideal outcome, if everything I believed was true, would be for Ellman to be struck off. The other problem with legal action would be proving my case. There was never going to be a blood-soaked swab or sponge. If there ever had been one, it had been quietly disposed of long ago. The evidence I had to support my beliefs was circumstantial. Nothing was clear-cut, and although in civil actions I knew a case could be won on the balance of probability, I still did not rate my chances very highly. If I brought an action and lost it, the consequences would be dire. I would have to meet my own legal fees and those of the other side. Financially, it could wipe me out. We could even lose the house, and that would not be fair on Mike. I didn't want to add poverty to my list of woes, and at my time of life, and in my state of health, there would be no possibility of rectifying such a disastrous situation. So for the time being, I would have to rule out legal action.

I was not so much at a crossroads as up a cul-de-sac. Was there a way out? What else could I do? I wondered how closed the medical ranks really were. I suspected that a number of doctors at Casterbridge Hospital had inevitably been drawn into the cover-up. Dr Hick's loyalty was already suspect. Dr Kemp, probably the most junior member of the team, had struck me as nervous, and liable to let things slip. Other consultants had been involved. And what about the four partners in my GP's practice? I suspected they knew quite a lot. Should I target anyone in particular?

After a lot of thought, I decided to write individual letters to the consultant radiologist who had decided in October 2000 that the unidentified mass did not need treatment, to the radiographer who had done the ultrasound scan which had identified the mass, to the bowel consultant who had carried out a sigmoidoscopy before the September 2000 operation, and to Dr Hick, who had now moved to another hospital, sensible woman.

The letters were similar in nature, in that all explained the mental anguish I was suffering as a consequence of the confusion and uncertainty surrounding my medical condition. There were then specific questions which I felt were relevant for the various specialists. I asked the consultant radiologist about his understanding of the nature of the mass, and whether it could naturally shrink away. I also asked why he thought Ellman had not passed my case to him after the February 2000 operation when the histology had shown borderline cancer. I asked the radiographer about the term 'recurrent ovarian cancer' which he had used in his scan report of August 2000. Did he mean recurrent from 1981, or recurrent from February 2000? Had my 1981 cancer been cured, which is what I had always been led to believe? The bowel specialist was simply asked what he thought is/was wrong with me. I reminded him about his suggestion of a haematoma obstructing my bowel, but pointed out that surely Ellman would have recognised one, and would have told me about it.

The letter to Dr Hick was much longer. Of all my contacts in the medical profession, I felt that she was the one most likely to squeal, especially now that she had left Casterbridge Hospital. She, more than any of the others, had tried to convey to me that something was very wrong. I already knew she wanted to tell me something. The problem was, would she dare to blow the whistle? There was also the fact that she was a woman. This could make her more sympathetic towards me, and, depending on her personal circumstances, mean that she might be less concerned than a man would be about jeopardising her career. I began the letter with 'I have a feeling you might remember me'. Of course she would! If everything I believed was true, the matter would constantly prey on her mind. I thanked her for her care in September 2000, and assured her that I was still in good health. I then went on to explain that both in September 2000 and February 2001 I had been aware, because of her prolonged eye contact, that she was trying to tell me something. I suggested that she had been due to see me in February 2001, but had passed me on to Ellman because she did not want to lie to me if I asked awkward questions. Had she deliberately and untruthfully told him I was with my husband, which suggested there could be trouble? I told her that Ellman had written in my file that I had left with my husband. I then went on to tell her about my findings regarding the fabricated histology report and the forged back-up documents. It was only fair to make her aware of the possible extent of Ellman's misconduct. She would have to decide what, if anything, she was going to do about it, and I acknowledged that I had put her in a moral dilemma.

It was now the end of March 2002. This time there would be no long wait for reports. Responses, if there were any, would arrive within two or three weeks. But rather than wait doing nothing, I decided to pursue another course of action. The handwriting report had added considerable evidence to the possibility that medical documents in my file had been fabricated and forged. It was time to go back to the police. This time I did not simply walk into the local police station. Instead I wrote to the forgery department at the county headquarters, hoping in that way to get straight to the right specialist. The letter was quite short. I mentioned my earlier contact with the police, and the investigations I had made since then, including the report on the handwriting. As the matter was very complicated, I asked for an interview with an officer specialising in forgery.

This did not take place until the 16th of April, which, as it happened, was fortunate, because at the beginning of April I became very ill with a chest infection. I went to the surgery on a Saturday morning and saw the only doctor on duty, the most junior partner. She prescribed me some antibiotics, but by the Monday morning I was worse, feeling too ill to get out of bed. Mike phoned the surgery and requested a home visit. To our utter amazement Dr Foyle was at the door about twenty minutes later. Most doctors conduct their morning surgeries before making home visits unless it is an emergency. I was certainly very ill, but I was not dying. Mike showed him up to the bedroom and hovered outside the door. I hadn't seen Dr Foyle since the breakdown of my relationship with Ellman. I wondered if he had been informed of this, and whether he would take the opportunity to check my abdomen and suggest I should see another gynaecologist.

He seemed in a great hurry. He listened to my chest through his stethoscope, identified an infection low down in my left lung, and prescribed some stronger antibiotics.

"Should I stay in bed?" I asked, rather hoping I might have an excuse to expect Mike to wait on me hand and foot.

"No. Get up, move around a bit, and sit in a chair," he advised.

With that he was gone, as if he couldn't get out of the place fast enough. So, not even a passing enquiry about gynaecological matters. That was not necessarily because he was not aware of the situation, I surmised. It could have been because he knew there was nothing to be concerned about, or it could have been because he found the whole scenario so embarrassing that he did not want the matter raised, which would explain why he had dashed out so fast. It might also explain why he had come so quickly. Perhaps he did not want one of his partners, possibly the one taking house calls that day, to see me. Perhaps he did not trust them to handle the matter the way he would want. I sank back on the pillows and thought about everything in a very feverish and muddle-headed way.

A few days later a letter arrived from Casterbridge Hospital. It was from the patient liaison manager. The consultant radiologist I had written to had passed the letter to her with instructions that he could not answer my queries because the matter had been the subject of my complaint against Ellman. It was suggested I discuss matters with my GP. None of the other doctors I had written to responded. That didn't surprise me. I felt sure that most of them suspected something even if they were not fully in the picture. But they were not going to reveal anything. They wanted a quiet life, and who could blame them? Doing nothing was obviously the best course of action. My letters would have been hastily binned. Why the radiologist had acted differently, I could not imagine. Perhaps he felt he might have a closer personal involvement in the matter.

The letter to the police headquarters resulted in an interview with Detective Sergeant Kirk Langley. I had typed out a statement giving brief details of my medical history up to November 2000. I then added that I believed that Ellman had attempted to persuade his colleagues to give me chemotherapy by fabricating the 1981 histology report and placing it with my notes in a way to make it appear it was related to the February 2000 investigations. In response to my complaints and inquiries, back-up documents had been forged. I suggested that the hospital administrators could have been involved as well as Ellman.

In a further statement I explained why I thought Ellman was guilty of criminal acts and how I had suffered as a victim of these acts. I pointed out that there was a criminal element to the case because I believed that Ellman had deliberately followed a course of action to cover up his negligence which had caused me unnecessary suffering. I mentioned that I endured six months of impaired bowel movements and had then had to have a further operation which meant at least a month of convalescence. Mentally, I had had to cope with an on-off cancer diagnosis, as had all my friends and relatives. The confusion had caused me terrible anxiety, and I suggested that it was only my firm beliefs and strength of character which had prevented me from having a nervous breakdown. I pointed out how Ellman had dragged other doctors into the cover-up, and concluded that he was a disgrace to his profession, and that to protect the well-being of other women in Casterbridge, he should be suspended while matters were investigated.

I felt I had prepared quite thoroughly for the interview. Mike and I and the Detective Sergeant sat round the dining room table while I went through everything. It took about forty minutes. DS Langley made some notes, asked a few questions in areas where he was not clear about events, and then said he would decide what further enquiries to make. He warned us that it might take some while, but at least it seemed he was taking the matter seriously. Perhaps, through the rather indirect route of investigating the forgery, we might get somewhere. There was no way I was giving up.

CHAPTER 10

The late spring of 2002 was a very unusual time in the Casterbridge area. There was murder after murder, quite unprecedented for a quiet and reasonably affluent area on the south coast. It was more like the fictitious Oxford inhabited by Chief Inspector Morse. The police must have been stretched almost beyond limit, and, quite rightly, my case must have been put on the back burner.

Firstly there was a delay while the police obtained my records from the hospital. That took over a month, but at least they appeared to be taking the matter seriously and doing things thoroughly. Early in July I contacted DS Langley to ask him about progress on the case. He apologised for the delay, but I assured him I wasn't surprised in the circumstances. He said he was waiting to speak to Dr Appleyard, the pathologist who had apparently prepared the 1981 histology report, to ask him if it was his handwriting on the back-up document. I had never thought of tackling the case in that way, but I suppose it made sense. Presumably Langley had checked that Appleyard was still alive, although I suspected that as it was now twenty one years since he did the report, he was probably retired.

Then something very fortuitous happened. I suppose you would call it serendipity. One evening I was idly watching the local TV news while eating my tea. There had, possibly, been yet another murder. A decaying body had been found in suspicious circumstances in Titchmouth, the next large town along the coast. A Dr Appleyard, the forensic pathologist, was briefly shown striding away from the Coroner's office. I was immediately all eyes and ears. I saw a slim, athletic-looking man who could not have been a day over fifty, probably younger. If he was now a forensic pathologist he would certainly be very well known and respected by all police officers in the area. No doubt Langley was anxious to ensure that a document carrying his name was above-board. But what if it wasn't? I imagined that if anyone had misused Appleyard's name, the police would be down on them like a ton of bricks.

Then another point occurred to me. Dr Appleyard appeared too young to have been a consultant in 1981. I assumed he was now fifty. He would have been born in 1952. Assuming he had gone straight to medical school on leaving secondary education after 'A' levels, he would have completed his medical training at the age of twenty-five in 1977. Then he would have gone through the usual junior and senior houseman posts before becoming a registrar. At some stage he might have needed extra training when he had decided to specialise in pathology. Even if he was an exceptionally lucky high-flyer, he could not have been a consultant in June 1981. Surely that took at least six years?

I discussed this with my Scrabble friend, Amy. She had been a senior secretary at Casterbridge Hospital for many years, retiring in September 1981.

"The police are going to check that Appleyard, the pathologist, did actually write the handwritten histology report the hospital sent me. You know, a funny thing happened the other night. Appleyard was on the telly –the local news – about that body in Titchmouth."

"Appleyard?" Amy exclaimed. "I don't remember an Appleyard at Casterbridge Hospital. I'm sure I would have remembered an unusual name like that."

"He was the consultant pathologist in 1981," I told her. "That's the name on the histology report – Dr A Appleyard."

"In 1981 the consultant pathologist was a Dr Hewson. He's retired now, but I met him at a function a year or two ago."

Amy had kept up with many of her old colleagues through the hospital's retirement association, and for a woman of eighty-one, she was quite exceptionally physically and mentally active. I didn't doubt her memory for one minute.

"So there was no Appleyard at Casterbridge Hospital in 1981," I said.

"Definitely not," Amy replied in her precise manner.

"That doesn't entirely surprise me," I went on. "On the telly Appleyard didn't look old enough to be a consultant in 1981. I think Ellman just sort of used his name because he is well known and respected. There isn't any backup documentation with Appleyard's name on it."

"Perhaps back in '81 bits were sent to another hospital for analysis," Amy suggested. "A lot of that went on."

"I doubt it somehow. You've got to remember that Casterbridge was a major cancer centre even in 1981. Also, I got the result quickly – the op was on a Sunday, so the path lab would have started work on the Monday. I got the result early Friday morning, so the doctors probably got it during the Thursday."

"It's all a bit of a mystery," Amy concluded.

"I wonder what the police will find out?" I added.

While DS Langley was still faffing about, I thought how I might obtain a sample of Appleyard's handwriting. I found out from the Medical Register where he lived – right out in the countryside. Perhaps I could go to his house and ask him to sponsor me for something and write his name and address on a form. The trouble with that idea was that only school kids went round with sponsorship forms, and that it would probably be his wife or children who answered the door. What a stupid idea! I had to admit defeat. The matter was in the hands of the police, and that is where it would have to stay.

All the same, I continued with somewhat fanciful speculation about Appleyard. The entry in the Medical Register described him as a Home Office forensic pathologist. I got the impression he was very high-ranking. I wondered how many criminals were banged up as a result of his forensic evidence. He had to be a professional man of the utmost integrity, not only whiter than white, but seen to be so. I became increasingly convinced that he had nothing to do with the 1981 histology report, and that he was completely unaware of how his name had been used on the fabricated document. When DS Langley did finally manage to approach him, I could imagine him being utterly horrified. Casterbridge Hospital and Ellman would then be deep in the shit.

In fact, shit was increasingly on my mind – real shit, that is. During the early part of the summer my bowels had been periodically playing up, causing attacks of diarrhoea and the passing of mucus. At first I thought it was due to the antibiotics I had taken for the chest infection, because the leaflet with the pills had mentioned bowel disturbances as a possible side effect. Then I put it down to over-indulgence on seasonal fruit – I love both strawberries and cherries – but you can have too much of a good thing. However, the problem persisted. I was reluctant to go to the doctor because of the great uncertainty surrounding my pelvic condition, and the on-going police enquiry, which I felt sure was going to be the key which would open a festering can of worms.

By early August, after I had tried the usual over-the-counter cures for dodgy bowels without success, I decided I had to go to the doctor. I didn't want an appointment with Dr Foyle because I had become increasingly suspicious that he was somehow covering up for Ellman. Fortunately the first appointment available was with Dr Wilson, the second most senior partner in the four-partner practice.

I sat down beside his desk and described my symptoms. I also mentioned that the sigmoidoscopy report of September

2000 had mentioned some evidence of diverticular disease, and I suggested that this might be the cause of my problems. He found the report in my file and looked at it without comment. Next he had me up on the couch, feeling my abdomen and probing up my vagina.

"Is everything all right?" I asked.

"Seems to be," he replied.

Then it was over on my side so he could do a rectal examination.

"Is it all right?" I asked again as I slipped off the couch.

"Yes," he said in a rather absent-minded way. He looked very puzzled. I tried to fathom out what was on his mind, but couldn't. However, something was troubling him.

We sat down at the desk again. He asked about my recent medical history.

"I had my left ovary removed along with a cyst, and a sub-total hysterectomy in February 2000. Then another lump developed, so in September 2000 I had another op, but Ellman said he couldn't remove it. But I think he did do something because I had bowel problems then, but they got better quickly after the op. It's very confusing..."

At that point I dried up. I just didn't know what to say. I'd voiced the official line, and added a little about my doubts. What more could I do? Dr Wilson frowned and started flipping through my file.

"I think I'll have to read through your notes before I decide on what's to be done," he said. "I'll phone you in a day or two."

I left the surgery. Something was going on, I just knew it. Dr Wilson was being so cautious. He had started off acting quite normally, but after the rectal examination he had suddenly changed. Was it because he had felt something very odd, or was it because he had suddenly remembered something? I had been fairly sure all along that Dr Foyle had briefed his partners about the cover-up, if, indeed, one had been going on. But that was now over two years ago, and a busy GP like Dr Wilson would have forgotten about it, until my presence had jogged his memory. Yes, that's what must have happened. Dr Wilson, as well as reading my notes, would be having frantic discussions with Dr Foyle as to how he should proceed. I tried to imagine I was a fly on the wall...

Wilson: "I had Mrs Bland in the surgery today. She's got bowel symptoms - diarrhoea, mucus."

Foyle: "Monica Bland? Bloody hell!"

Wilson: "Exactly. I remembered something halfway through the consultation, but couldn't quite recall the details. So I said I'd have to read her notes and phone her. Fortunately she didn't give me any trouble, but I think she's a bit suspicious about things."

Foyle: "I'm damn sure she is. She's not thick, and neither is her husband. You know she's been on to the GMC, and then she went through the NHS complaints system, without success. Ellman's kept me updated."

Wilson: "So it's to do with Ellman, not us."

Foyle: "Well, not directly."

Wilson: "Meaning what?"

Foyle: "We've been aware of what's been going on, haven't we?"

Wilson: "Remind me of the details. I can't remember, and I assume there won't be anything in the file, will there?"

Foyle: "Ellman botched the first op, put things right in the second op, but made out that was necessary because another cyst had developed."

Wilson: "Botched? In what way?"

Foyle: "He's always been a bit vague on that point. I honestly don't know. But it was the plan that things would be put right by a second op, and that we were expected to hold the fort meanwhile. I definitely remember telling you and the others about that."

Wilson: "Yes, I do remember something, and I remember

being very unhappy about how we'd been dragged into the mess. And now it seems everything is flaring up again, and what's worse, we've got a suspicious patient now."

Foyle: "You're going to have to be careful."

Wilson: "Me! We all are. You know she seems to flit between all of us. Everyone's got to be briefed. We've got to have a plan. And we've got to do something. There *is* something wrong with her and given her history, it could be cancer."

Foyle: "It's no great problem. Just refer her to the hospital, but not to Ellman, to the other one, what's his name."

Wilson: "Harcourt. But will she go? She doesn't seem to trust them at Casterbridge. She'll want to go to Titchmouth, or somewhere. Then some other guy will start digging into her notes and will smell a rat. Goodness knows what could happen!"

Foyle: "Refer her to Harcourt. You can trust him. Tell her it's urgent. Tell her Harcourt specialises in gynae cancers, which is true. But don't let her go anywhere else."

Wilson: "I don't like this."

Foyle: "Do you think I do?"

I had always regarded Foyle and Wilson as decent, competent, and hard-working GPs. Because of Ellman, they now found themselves in a terrible dilemma. There would be confusion about my condition, quite probably resulting in uncertainty as to how I should be treated. My care would definitely be compromised. Then there was the problem that the police enquiry was still on-going.

Two days later Dr Wilson phoned me.

"I've been through your notes. You have this mass," he said.

"Do I? Ellman said it was reactive swelling which was going away naturally."

"I don't think so. It could be cancerous. It's very important things are investigated properly. You need to see a specialist. Personally I think you need a CA125 blood test, an ultrasound scan, and a sigmoidoscopy."

"I'll have the blood test."

"Good. We can do that here in the surgery."

"But I want to consult someone privately, outside the area. I'm not happy about going back to Casterbridge Hospital because I made complaints about my previous treatment there."

"I wouldn't refer you to Ellman."

"I'm sure he wouldn't want to see me again. But I wouldn't trust his colleagues. They're all in it together."

"Consultants act completely independently," Dr Wilson tried to assure me. Crap, I thought. Not if it meant landing a colleague in the shit.

"I want to make my own arrangements," I said. "I know someone in the right field."

"I suggest you think about things. Meanwhile I'm going to contact another consultant at the hospital to see what he suggests. "I'll phone you again in a day or two."

"OK. 'Bye."

I slammed down the phone. I hadn't been lying when I said I knew someone in the right field. Mike and I had already discussed the matter. Over the years Mike's accountancy practice had gradually developed a specialisation in medical and dental accounting, and one of his ex-clients (he was now retired) was a lady gynaecologist with a very lucrative private practice. This Mary Tiller practiced well outside the local area, so would probably not know Ellman. Mike was very keen that I should consult her privately, and that because of the personal contact, he felt sure she would see me without a referral from my GP. I wanted an assessment of my condition from someone without prior knowledge of my medical history, some of which, I believe, had been deliberately falsified. It was an extremely difficult and delicate situation in which to find oneself. That I should develop new symptoms before the investigation into Ellman was completed, was something I'd been dreading. Now, it seemed, this nightmare was reality.

The following day, before I had definitely decided on any course of action, Dr Wilson phoned again.

"I've had a talk with Mr Harcourt at Casterbridge Hospital," he began. "He's a specialist in gynaecological cancers and he definitely thinks you need some urgent investigation. Have you thought about the situation since yesterday?"

"Yes, and I still want to see someone right outside the area, and I'm prepared to pay for it. I still have someone in mind whom I know personally." (In truth, I had never met Mary Tiller.)

"No consultant will see you without a referral from me. Whoever it is will also need to see your hospital notes and it could take time to get them transferred. And another thing, if you see someone privately, you'll then have to continue in the private sector."

His last point came as a surprise to me. I had always thought I could see a consultant privately but then elect to have any necessary treatment on the NHS. I knew of friends who had done this. In fact, I found out later I was right. I think Dr Wilson was doing everything he could to dissuade me from moving outside the sphere of influence of Casterbridge Hospital. His voice sounded slightly strange. It's well known that the phone can emphasise slight abnormalities in the voice or speech patterns. Perhaps that's because in the absence of visual signs one is more likely to be receptive to auditory signals. Yes, there definitely seemed to be a slight tremor in his voice, suggesting he was lying to me.

"All I want is an opinion from someone who has no knowledge of my previous medical history," I said, beginning to feel very confused as to what I did actually want.

"But that won't be possible," Dr Wilson explained. "Wherever you go, your notes go."

"I see." I was at a loss. Perhaps it would be a waste of time and money to see Mary Tiller. "I'll have to think about it," I concluded, "but meanwhile I'll have the CA125 blood test. If that's abnormal, we'll take it from there."

"That's fine. The practice nurse can do that. I'll put you through to reception for an appointment. But do give some thought to things because it's pretty obvious to me that you need further investigation and treatment."

I promised him that I would, and made arrangements for a blood sample to be taken. Poor Dr Wilson. I knew he was trying to do his best for me, but he must have found my attitude somewhat puzzling. Just how much did he know about the cover-up? What did he think I knew? He must have been thinking that if he wasn't careful he'd be dragged into the sorry affair. If only the police would get on with their enquiries into the forgery. If the slightest doubts were raised on that issue any doctor dealing with me would be most anxious to review my case and take absolutely nothing for granted.

I wanted to be open and honest with Dr Wilson. I wanted to tell him about my fears and suspicions, but with the police enquiry on-going, was this wise? I would ask DS Langley for advice, and I managed to contact him by phone. I explained about my declining health and the difficulties I was having with my GP. He admitted that he had still not contacted Dr Appleyard because he was a very difficult person to track down, but said he had no objection to me being open with my doctor.

I decided to write to Dr Wilson, as I could not possibly explain everything in the average five to ten minute appointment time. Sitting at my word processor forced me to think clearly and deal with events in the right order. Then I could review what I'd written and make any necessary changes. Dr Wilson would then have everything clearly in writing, so would not have to rely on his own scribbled consultation notes.

My letter began "I know you are doing your best to help me and I appreciate that you must find my attitude somewhat strange." I went on to detail the confusing events surrounding my September 2000 operation and the subsequent consultation with Ellman. Then I explained how I had been through the complaints procedure with both the GMC and NHS to no avail, how I had written to doctors other than Ellman who had been involved with my case and had been met with a wall of silence, and how what I believed were forged and fabricated documents were now in the hands of Casterbridge CID. I even gave him Langley's name in case he wanted to pass on any knowledge. I had the feeling Dr Wilson was an exceptionally decent guy who might, possibly, be tempted to whistle-blow if, indeed, he was aware of a cover-up. I enclosed a sample of my faeces which I asked him to send to the hospital lab to see whether or not my problems were due to a bowel infection. I handed in the letter when I went to the surgery for my blood test.

I received the result of the test during a consultation with Dr Wilson in early September. It was 165, which was high, bearing in mind that a normal reading was anything under 30. It was far higher than the 95 it had been before my February 2000 operation. Obviously something was going seriously wrong. Mike had come with me on this occasion, partly because I wanted a witness if Dr Wilson made any interesting comments about the content of my recent letter, and partly because, I believe, he was concerned about my reluctance to seek further treatment. Mike didn't say anything during the consultation, but I could feel he was willing me to put everything else to one side and concentrate entirely on the present situation. It seemed I had no choice.

"I really think you should see Mr Harcourt as soon as possible," Dr Wilson said.

"Yes, I suppose I must," I heard myself saying.

"I'll fast-track you. You should get an appointment in about two weeks."

Once we'd left the surgery I made it clear to Mike that I was very unhappy about the situation.

"I don't like the idea of going back to Casterbridge Hospital," I said. "OK, I'm seeing a different consultant, but he'll have discussed my case with Ellman and will have been fed a load of bullshit. He'll have a completely distorted view of what's going on."

"I think you'll find consultants, even those in the same hospital, make up their own mind about things," Mike replied, trying to reassure me. "If this Harcourt thinks Ellman has made mistakes, he won't say anything to you, but he will do what he considers best for you. You think about it, he won't want to be dragged into the mess, will he?"

"Huh! I don't trust these doctors. They're far more concerned about protecting each other than doing what's best for the patient."

Once more I was faced with the question of how far a doctor would risk his own career to protect a colleague.

"Anyway, you will see Harcout, won't you," Mike urged. "You can't go on as you are."

Mike was right. The bowel problems were getting worse, and I was having to rush to the loo about every two hours, day and night. I was also getting pains in the pelvic area, and generally felt a bit under the weather. No medication, either over-the-counter, or from the doctor, made any difference. Tests on the faeces showed no bowel infection. My problems were almost certainly due to a lump pressing on the bowel.

On the 18th of September DS Langley phoned. At last he had been able to ask Dr Appleyard if the writing on the back-up documents to the fabricated histology report was his. Dr Appleyard informed him that he had written the first paragraph, and that the second paragraph, which was in a different hand, would have been written by his assistant taking dictated notes from him. Therefore DS Langley regarded the investigation as completed.

Another blow. Another dead end. However, I was less deflated than I thought I would have been. I had a feeling that Langley had not seen Dr Appleyard. He had just wanted to get rid of the case, and I had been fobbed of with false information. I would make my own enquiries. I began by writing to the Royal College of Pathologists requesting brief details of the positions held by Dr Alec Appleyard since he qualified in 1977.

CHAPTER 11

I was becoming increasingly suspicious about every aspect of my case, and when Mike and I saw Mr Harcourt on the 26th of September, I had a small cassette recorder hidden in my bag. Perhaps Mr Harcourt would let something slip about Ellman. If so, I wanted it preserved as possible evidence. I knew what these consultants were like – they'd quite happily deny what I had clearly heard them say. Ellman had quite clearly used the phrase 'reactive swelling' but had gone on to deny it. What a pity I hadn't taped him.

I had also prepared a brief summary of events since February 2000, including things that had appeared to go wrong, and the inconsistences in my treatment under Ellman. I even included my own suspicions about the 'foreign object' scenario. I felt it was only right that Mr Harcourt should be aware of my view of events.

During the usual half-hour or so wait beyond my appointment time, I was approached by the drippy Natalie, the Macmillan nurse. Despite the fact that she hadn't seen me for over two and a half years, she remembered me. No doubt my name on some appointment list had jogged her memory, but I suspected that it might have been something else as well that had lodged my name firmly in her mind.

"How are you?" she asked, sitting down on the bench beside me.

"Huh! Back here, aren't I," was by brief reply. She touched my arm lightly in the way these people are probably trained to do.

"So you're having more problems," she prompted.

"I keep having diarrhoea. The doctor thinks there's a lump pressing on the bowel."

Her drippy ways hadn't changed at all. She looked at me with rather soulful eyes, like a dog wanting its dinner when it wasn't feeding time.

"Remember I'm always here if you need me. Do you have my phone number?"

"Yes, I do." I remembered seeing the leaflet she had given me in 2000 tucked away in my 'medical matters' file.

Eventually we were shown into Mr Harcourt's consulting room. Mike accompanied me, as did Natalie. There was also another nurse present, so the room was quite crowded. Mr Harcourt obviously thought he needed two witnesses. I was glad I had Mike with me and that my tape recorder was now running silently in my bag. It seemed that protecting/ uncovering the cover-up was of greater importance to both sides than my current state of health. I still have the tape, so here are some relevant extracts.

Harcourt: "Dr Wilson rang me up and wrote a letter explaining things. We've not met before, have we?"

Me: "No."

Harcourt: "Let's start at the beginning. How old are you?"

Me: "I'm fifty-six now."

Harcourt: "And are you working now?"

Me: "No, I'm retired."

Harcourt: "Have you had children?"

Me: "No."

Harcourt: "Now, you've had a hysterectomy...."

Me: "I had a sub-total hysterectomy in February 2000 as part of the operation to remove an ovarian cyst on my left ovary. As far as I'm aware the only things left now are a little bit of womb, my cervix, and vagina."

Harcourt: "What symptoms are you getting at the moment?"

Me: "Purely bowel symptoms. About the beginning of June I

got some slight diarrhoea symptoms. These kept coming and going, and since early August have been here all the time. It's pretty watery with mucus and I have to go about every couple of hours.

Harcourt: "Any pain?"

Me: "Yes, I get diarrhoea type pains, you know, cramping pain sometimes, not all the time. I take aspirin, which helps. I've tried other things like Immodium and codeine phosphate but they haven't had any effect."

Harcourt: "Are you losing weight?"

Me: "No. My weight seems to be steady. In fact, I'm nearly a stone heavier than I was two years ago."

Harcourt: "And you're eating all right?"

Me: "Yes, but I'm tending to avoid richer things which I feel might upset me more, but generally I'm eating normally."

Harcourt: "Are the water works normal?"

Me: "Yes, but as it seems natural to empty my bladder when I empty my bowels, I go quite often."

Harcourt: "You had your appendix out..."

Me: "I never had my appendix out." (Thought; what sort of a mess are my notes in?)

Harcourt: "You had your right ovary out in 1981."

Me: "That's right. Why you thought I had my appendix out was because I came in expecting to have my appendix out, but when they opened me up they found it wasn't my appendix – it was cancer of the ovary."

Harcourt: "And you had radiotherapy to the pelvis after that."

Me: "That's right, under Dr Carson, an excellent chap."

Harcourt: "Then in 1999 another mass was found, and Mr Ellman did the hysterectomy, and took out the left ovary."

Me: "Yes, that's right."

Harcourt: "And were things all right after that?"

Me: "Not entirely, because some rather odd things happened. A month after the op I had a watery discharge, and pain for about a week, which I wasn't expecting. I went to the doctor and she phoned Mr Ellman who said it was normal, but why wasn't I told to expect it? I'd had virtually no discharge just after the operation. Then after the discharge stopped I started getting bowel problems. I could only pass rabbit-size motions, quite a lot of mucus, quite frequent, not the same as I've got now but I didn't have pain with it because it wasn't really diarrhoea. Then the scan showed a mass pressing on the bowel, which probably explained why I had the problems."

Harcourt: "Yes, OK."

Me: "After the second operation, after which I was informed nothing was done, the bowel problem cleared up within a couple of weeks. Then for about twenty months my bowels were normal which for me is going twice, occasionally even three times a day."

Harcourt: "Now could I examine you?"

Natalie showed me into the adjoining examination room. I took care to take my bag with the cassette recorder in it, and Mike came too. I took off my trousers and briefs and Natalie got me settled on the couch, trying to get me relaxed by talking about my recent holiday in Scotland. Then Mr Harcourt came in and pressed all over my abdomen, finding a tender spot very low down. Then the dreaded words:

Harcourt: "Can I just check below? There's definitely a lump there."

That meant a prod up the vagina. He pulled on a latex glove and lubricated a finger while I gritted my teeth.

Me: "Dr Wilson said everything felt nice and soft."

Harcourt: (poking around) "Is that tender there?"

Me: "I'm not sure – I just generally don't like internal examinations."

Harcourt: "That bit – is that tender?"

Me: "No, not more than anywhere else."

Harcourt: (withdrawing his finger) "OK. There is this mass there. I think it's pushing the bowel backwards, probably causing the diarrhoea. Er, I think what we need is a thing called a cat scan and have a look to see what else is going on and have a chat after that."

Me: "Is the high CA125 test significant?"

Harcourt: "Possibly. It can be raised by a whole lot of things, some of them quite normal."

Me: "Perhaps by my bowels being upset?"

Harcourt: "Yes."

Me; "Is this a completely new thing?"

Harcourt: "I suspect not. I suspect it's related to the lumps you had two years ago, which they say they couldn't remove. But I'm hoping the scan will shed some light on exactly what it is and where it is, and then we can advise you on how to treat it."

Me: "Would it be surgically?"

Harcourt: "I don't know at this stage. Perhaps it would be with drugs. Right, I'll arrange for a cat scan."

Me: "Not an ultrasound scan?" (I remembered in Ellman's submission to the GMC that he had claimed ultrasound scans were suitable for monitoring my condition.)

Harcourt: "Definitely a cat scan."

I put my clothes on again and we all returned to the consulting room. I was given a form to take to the X-ray department for an urgent cat (or CT) scan. Before I left I briefly explained that basically I had had two versions of my condition after the September 2000 operation, one being that the lump had gone naturally, and one that it was still there. I gave Mr Harcourt the summary of all my suspicions which I had printed on pink paper so that it stood out, and asked him to place it in my file. I also indicated that I wanted to put the matter behind me, and that my principal concern was to get better. I think Mike was relieved to hear me saying that, and to a large extent I meant it. However, my enquiries were still on-going, and I wasn't giving up while there were still avenues to pursue.

So we left the consulting room none the wiser about any possible wrong-doing in the past. I had been quite impressed by Mr Harcourt. He had been polite, pragmatic, and thorough. If only I had been referred to him in 2000. I should have been, seeing I had a previous history of ovarian cancer, and he was the local specialist in that area. However, I did feel he was treading very carefully. I think he knew something, and he now had the difficult task of treating me as best he could without doing anything which might open a seething can of worms. I didn't envy him.

"I think you're in good hands now," Mike said as we made our way home. "I suggest you try and put everything behind you and just concentrate on getting well again."

"I suppose you're right," I agreed reluctantly. "But what worries me is that there's been a false medical history created for me, and that this could effect how they treat me."

"I think Harcourt's very much his own man. He'll work from how things are now. He probably won't pay too much attention to what's gone on in the past."

While waiting for the CT scan, I heard from the Royal College of Pathologists. Apparently they were not able to give me information about Dr Appleyard because it would be in breach of the Data Protection Act. Yet again I had reached a dead-end. I decided to write back to the Chief Executive of the College with the full story of the fabricated documents and the police enquiry. The angle I took was that Ellman had probably used Dr Appleyard's name in an illegal and possibly damaging way, and that therefore the matter should be investigated further. I explained why I believed Dr Appleyard had never been a consultant at Casterbridge Hospital. I also suggested that it was possible that the police had not made proper enquiries. I pointed out that someone of Dr Appleyard's standing would never actually be involved in creating false documents, and neither would he lie to protect a colleague. I also included details of the handwriting expert's report, which strongly suggested the back-up documents had been created by Ellman and his junior. I awaited the reply with interest.

On the 3rd of October I had a CT scan. It was all quite complicated. Firstly I had to drink a litre of some foul-tasting fruit squash which had something in it that would make my innards show up on the scan. Then I was moved backwards and forwards through a rather noisy ring doughnut-shaped piece of equipment. Then I was injected with some kind of contrast dye which made my bum feel hot, and was passed back and forth through the doughnut yet again. It all took ages and probably cost a lot. I could understand why doctors ordered ultrasound scans if they though they would be sufficient.

I saw Mr Harcourt again on the 17th of October. Once more Mike came with me, but the cassette recorder did not. I had concluded that nothing was going to be unintentionally revealed, and I wasn't happy with the subterfuge involved in secret recording. The drippy Natalie was hovering around again, and just her presence suggested the news was going to be bad.

Mr Harcourt explained that the CT scan showed a lump pressing on the rectum, and it was this that was causing the constant diarrhoea.

"It's grown about a centimetre since the last scan in August 2000," he said, perusing the scan report. "So it's very slow-growing. It's also likely to be difficult or impossible to remove. If it couldn't be removed two years ago, I wouldn't be happy trying again. It could mean you having a permanent colostomy."

"I don't want that," I replied with horror.

"I'm sure you don't if it can be avoided. But there's something else we can try. There's an experimental treatment you can have at Titchmouth. I couldn't say how effective it might be...."

"But it could be worth a try, better than having yet another operation."

"So you'd like to try it?"

"Yes. If it doesn't work, then I suppose we'll have to think about surgery."

"I'll refer you to my colleague, Dr Oswald. He can tell you far more about this treatment. Natalie, could you arrange for Mrs Bland to have an urgent appointment with Dr Oswald."

Natalie slipped down from her perch on top of a cupboard in the crowded little room and filled in a form.

Now I had to ask the question which had been uppermost in my mind for months.

"Is it cancer?"

Mr Harcourt seemed to hesitate. He looked at the scan report again. "I can't tell."

"But what about the high CA125 reading?" I prompted him.

Once again he seemed uncertain. "It doesn't look good," he finally concluded.

So Mike and I went home still not really knowing what was wrong with me. Perhaps this Dr Oswald would shed more light on the matter.

"I just can't believe this lump has been there all the time," I said. "It seems they think it rapidly grew from nothing to about nine centimetres between the ops in 2000, and then over the next two years just grew by another centimetre or so. Or it may not have gown at all. Perhaps the CT scan is just more accurate than the ultrasound."

"It does all seem rather odd," Mike agreed.

"I'm sticking to my foreign object scenario. This present lump is new, and this time it's home-gown, as it were. I reckon it started growing in the spring when I first started to notice occasional bowel problems, you know, mucus, a bit loose. Surely if the lump had been there all the time, I'd have had these symptoms all the time."

"I'm inclined to agree with you."

"But they're treating me as if I've got some kind of slow-growing lump. Probably they think it's cancer. I reckon this treatment in Titchmouth is some form of chemotherapy, only for some reason they won't use the word. But nine or ten centimetres is very large for a cancer tumour. You'd think that by now it would have spread and that I'd be quite ill generally."

"But you're reasonably OK except for your bowels."

"Exactly. I reckon it's some kind of cyst again. That's why it's so big and why it's grown so quickly. But for them to accept that, it means they've got to own up to what's gone on in the past, and they're not going to do that, are they?"

"It's a very difficult situation," Mike agreed.

Except for being there, and being generally sympathetic, Mike was of little use. He was as lost and confused as I was.

"But this CA125 reading is worrying," Mike went on. "It seems that is a sign of cancer. You can't afford not to do anything."

"I know I can't. But back in 2000 they told me that infections can raise this CA125, so perhaps that's what's happening now. Perhaps I've got some pelvic infection caused by the cyst. And another thing, in September 2000 the CA125 was only 35, but the lump was nearly as big then. I don't reckon you can tell much from the CA125."

I was quite surprised at how bullish I had become. Perhaps it was just an elaborate way of burying my head in the sand, but at least it was better than becoming depressed and giving up. I had always known that when it came to cancer, if, indeed, that was what it was, a positive mental attitude was vital. I wasn't going to give up either on my own health, or on trying to find out what had gone on in 2000. I was awaiting a reply from the Royal College of Pathologists with great interest. What would they make of the fabricated documents? I felt that these were now my only way back into the case. Mike read a lot of books on true crime, and he was always telling me that criminals were often found out because of inattention to some little detail, or because the investigators picked up on the significance of some apparently minor point. That was how Shipman had been exposed. The daughter of one of his victims noticed that he had forged a will. Soon after that the flood-gates opened. Perhaps the fabricated documents would be Ellman's undoing.

CHAPTER 12

I received a very prompt appointment to see Dr Oswald, and on the morning of the 23rd of October, Mike and I were shown into his consulting room. He appeared quite young, and unlike most consultants, he wore a spotless white coat.

He began by conveying Natalie's apologies for her absence. She had told me the previous week when she had arranged the appointment, that she would be at the clinic that day, and would be around if I needed her. (That had sounded ominous.) So it turned out that Mike and I were alone with Dr Oswald, which was a bit unusual. At all my previous consultations there had been a nurse present.

Dr Oswald began by explaining that the mass was very slow-growing and non-aggressive which apparently made it difficult to treat successfully. I must admit I found that rather difficult to understand. We then went on to discuss the experimental treatment Mr Harcourt had mentioned. It was called Octeotride, and Dr Oswald was quick to stress that it might not be effective. I had many questions about the nature of the treatment, and was told it would be given by injection every two or three weeks, and that serious side-effects were unlikely. That didn't sound too bad, but I knew enough to realise that we were talking about a form of chemotherapy, suggesting that the problem was indeed cancer. What had Dr Oswald deduced that Mr Harcourt hadn't? After all, they were both specialists in closely related areas, and they must have already discussed my case together. Why weren't they being open with me?

"I'd like to try this treatment," I said.

"Right, but first of all we'll have to see if your cells are compatible to ensure that the treatment will be beneficial."

"So you'll be wanting a biopsy of the lump."

"No, that won't be necessary. We'll use the samples obtained in February 2000."

"But that was nearly three years ago. Won't things have changed?"

"No, the 2000 samples will be fine," Dr Oswald assured me. Once more I felt very confused. The pathology in 2000 had only shown some cells having borderline changes, which could hardly be classed as cancer. Possibly things were a bit more advanced now. A biopsy struck me as very important in the circumstances.

"Now, there are other things we can do at the same time while you're being assessed for the Octeotride," Dr Oswald went on. "We must try to deal with your symptoms. I'll arrange for you to see Dr Keller who'll help you with your pain and bowel symptoms. Would you be happy with that?"

"Yes."

"Now the other possible thing we could do is refer you to Professor Shaw up at the City and Royal in London. He's just about the top gynaecological surgeon."

"So you think he could completely remove the lump?"

"I couldn't honestly say, but he's very highly regarded."

I wasn't going to pass up the opportunity of a referral to a top London surgeon. Anything to distance myself from Casterbridge Hospital and Ellman.

"I certainly think it would be worth getting his opinion," I replied. "What if he could remove the lump? Would that be a cure for the problem?"

"Oh no, it would just buy you some time. In a year or so you'd be back to square one. So it might not be worth having another operation. I'm afraid your cancer is incurable."

A sudden chill seemed to grip my whole body. I thought I

might faint. I glanced at Mike. He had gone as white as a sheet and seemed to have aged ten years in ten seconds. No doubt he could see a similar effect on me.

"No one's ever told me that before," I managed to mutter.

"Oh, I thought you knew," Dr Oswald replied, rather too breezily for my liking. As someone who was probably used to conveying bad news to his patients, his manner was remarkably unsympathetic. I felt my initial shock fading rapidly. Something was wrong; there was either a dreadful mix-up, or a deliberate cover-up, and I strongly suspected the latter. Sitting there, in a state of shock and confusion, I was unable to get my head around things. But one thing stood out – the sooner I got my care away from Casterbridge, the better. If anyone was going to start from scratch in assessing me, it would be a professor at a renowned teaching hospital.

"I'd still like to see Professor Shaw," I said.

"OK," Dr Oswald said as he scribbled notes in my file. "So the plan is this – referral to Professor Shaw, a consultation with Dr Keller, and assessment of cells for Octeotride. Now is there anything else you want to ask me?"

Initially my mind was a blank. I felt that I had many questions, but somehow I couldn't formulate them. What's more, I didn't trust Dr Oswald, or anyone else in Casterbridge Hospital for that matter. Somehow I managed to mentally click into gear.

"You say this lump is slow-growing?"

"Yes."

"So how come it appeared so quickly and grew so big between the February and September 2000 ops?"

"That probably wasn't the case. It would have been there by the first op."

"So Ellman missed it."

"He must have done," Dr Oswald conceded.

I hoped that the utter contempt I felt in my mind was reflected on my face. How could any surgeon miss a lump the size of a large orange? I simply didn't believe this strange scenario the doctors seemed to have concocted among themselves. I stuck with my own 'foreign object' scenario.

"Well, I'll make the necessary arrangements," Dr Oswald said. "You should get an appointment with Dr Keller and the City and Royal quite quickly."

Once we were out of the hospital and walking to where we had parked in a nearby back street, I started ranting and raving at Mike. Once again I was surprised at how bullish and confrontational I was.

"I just can't believe it," I began. "One week a consultant says he can't tell whether or not I've got cancer, then a week later another consultant says I've got incurable cancer. It beggars belief! They're all bloody useless!"

"It does seem rather odd," Mike agreed, looking grim.

"I reckon they're trying to write me off. You know, doctors like to bury their mistakes. I expect Ellman told Oswald I'd got incurable, inoperable cancer and that I should be left to die. They're like witch doctors in Africa - tell her she's going to die, and she will die. In Africa they point the bone or something. My aunt in Zimbabwe told me about it. It's the power of suggestion - only it won't work on me, because I don't trust them and I don't believe them."

"I think you're going a bit far," Mike cautioned.

"I'm not." I turned and looked at him as he puffed along, trying to keep up with me. "Don't tell me you actually believed what Oswald told us."

"He wouldn't lie about a thing like cancer. Doctors just wouldn't do that."

"Huh! I'd put nothing past them, the bastards. So you believe I've got incurable cancer."

"Well, it would seem like it. You've got to be sensible. You must go to see this professor."

"Don't worry, I will. It could be my one chance to get things sorted out."

I started to feel rather upset, not so much by the devastating diagnosis, which I honestly did not believe, but because Mike seemed to be siding with the doctors. That's all I needed.

"Why don't you go and see Terry Sutton again," Mike suggested. "See what he makes of it all."

"Yes, I will. Remind me to ring him when we get home."

We reached the car and I drove home in silence. Then as I backed up the drive a sudden thought came to me.

"What do I tell people?"

"Don't tell them anything," Mike replied. "Why upset them, perhaps unnecessarily?"

I looked at him. Was some element of doubt creeping into his mind?

As always, Terry managed to squeeze me into his packed schedule, and I saw him a week later. He carried out what he called bio-terrain tests on my blood, urine, and saliva. For once, it all seemed quite conventional. He looked at the acidity and alkalinity of these bodily fluids, and looked at my blood cells through a microscope. I even looked at them myself, although it didn't mean much to me.

"There are a lot of white blood cells," he explained. "This would indicate that your body is fighting something, but I don't think it's cancer. It could be an infection. I wouldn't like to say you haven't got cancer, but if you have it would seem it's in its early stages. Your body may be fighting it, and that could make you vulnerable to other infections. I'll do what I can to boost your immune system."

This was all slightly better news, and it made me suspect even more strongly that the cancer diagnosis had been based on the flimsiest of evidence, and that there was indeed an attempt being made by someone, somewhere, to get me labelled a hopeless case.

"Why couldn't the hospital do some more blood tests and things?" I asked. "All they've done is a CA125. That's up, so they assume its cancer, when they know damn well that there's a lot of other things that cause the CA125 to rise."

Terry shook his head. "Why a lot of things with the NHS.? They just seem to home in on the most likely diagnosis. They never look at the whole picture. They haven't got time."

Like most complimentary therapists, Terry believed strongly in a holistic approach, and was well aware that a minor problem in one part of the body could trigger problems elsewhere. He was relieved when I told him that I had had a troublesome tooth extracted.

Mike seemed quite relieved to hear Terry's verdict on the situation.

"It'll be interesting to see what the professor makes of it all," he mused.

"Yes. I should be getting an appointment any time now. I suppose I'm still being fast-tracked, which theoretically means I shouldn't have to wait more than two weeks for an appointment."

Two weeks passed, and I hadn't even received notification of an appointment, which I expected would give at least a week's notice of the actual appointment.

"That's the NHS for you," I said to Mike. "Why don't I just give up?" My constant pain and diarrhoea was really dragging me down, and somehow I could no longer summon up the energy to battle with the health service. But Mike was furious, and was becoming increasingly anxious about both my physical and mental state. He sat down at his computer and bashed out a really stroppy letter to the Chief Executive at Casterbridge Hospital, pointing out that as a cancer patient, I should get appointments within two weeks. To save time, he faxed the letter.

Two hours later Professor Shaw's secretary rang me offering me an appointment in just under two weeks. The following morning Dr Keller's secretary rang with an appointment in five days' time. At about the same time I received a letter from the hospital, dated the previous day, confirming that letters of referral had been sent to the appropriate consultants. Everything suggested that the Chief Executive had hit the panic button, and had personally got things moving. He was now trying to paper over whatever inefficiency it was that had caused the delay.

My suspicions deepened even further. I believed that the delay was nothing to do with administrative oversights. It was because Oswald and Ellman were having to contact Shaw and Keller to brief them on the cover-up. If the false medical history that had been created for me was to stay intact, it was important that everyone was singing from the same hymn sheet. If any new consultant was not prepared to play ball, I (I suspected) would not see him. But now the appointments had been made over the head of Oswald, so would I be seeing uncorrupted consultants? I doubted it. Frantic attempts would be made to ensure they were fully briefed, and even if Shaw and Keller were unhappy about the situation, they would almost certainly go along with it rather than spill the beans.

I was now deep into worst-possible-scenario territory. There was obviously something quite seriously wrong with me, but my problems were not being properly investigated because false assumptions were being made. No one was prepared to admit to this, because to do so would reveal a cover-up, which, unlike my cancer, had now reached massive proportions. What the hell could I do? There seemed to be two faint lights at the end of the tunnel. Perhaps Professor Shaw would cut through the crap, safe in the knowledge that his seniority, and the respect that he would have gained over the years, would protect him from any accusations of whistle-blowing. The other light was even fainter – legal action. I still felt I had insufficient evidence to mount a successful case, and knowing the speed at which the legal profession moved, I would be dead before I could prove anything.

CHAPTER 13

My letter to the Royal College of Pathologists containing details of the use of Dr Appleyard's name on fabricated documents had been sent on the 9th of October. Over a month had now passed, and I had not received a reply. Either the matter was being taken very seriously, or they were having some trouble in mixing a suitably opaque whitewash. Or was my letter simply being ignored? I concluded that I would have to find out by myself where Dr Appleyard had been working in the summer of 1981.

The Medical Register mentioned that he had previously been a Senior Registrar at Titchmouth, but no dates were included. There was nothing about a consultancy at Casterbridge. A friend found out quite a lot about him on the internet, but nothing about his previous appointments. Although the local library held copies of both the Medical Register and the Medical Directory, these were of no use for tracing a doctor's career. I needed the register for 1981, and the library did not keep old editions. But, I reasoned, the publishers of these tomes would certainly have back copies. As the Medical Directory seemed to give the most information on positions held, I wrote to the publishers asking for a copy of the entry for Dr Appleyard in the 1982 edition. (The information would have been collected in 1981.) Unfortunately the publishers had taken over the Medical Directory in 2000 and did not have access to previous editions. However, they told me that the British Medical Association held a complete set in their library, and helpfully provided contact details. I faxed the librarian and at last, on the 16th of November, I obtained the information I needed. The entry in the 1982 Medical Directory stated that Dr Appleyard was a Senior Registrar at Titchmouth General Hospital.

I now had evidence that the fabricated 1981 histology report included incorrect and deliberately misleading information. I was fairly sure that Dr Appleyard had not been involved in any way. The most likely explanation was that Ellman had deliberately added Appleyard's name because he needed to put some name, and had therefore chosen one which would have been both known, and held in high regard, by his colleagues. It was unfortunate that he had not thought to check whether or not Dr Appleyard had been a consultant in 1981.

I realised that the fabricated document was peripheral to my case. However, like the forged will in the Shipman case, it was a way in, something small which would lead on to greater things. I now felt more confident about embarking on legal action.

Neither Mike nor I had had much contact with the local legal profession. The obvious starting point was the firm who had handled our house conveyancing and will drafting, but they did not handle medical negligence. I trawled through the Yellow Pages, looking for an entry which specifically mentioned medical negligence. There was only one – Jeffreys and Rowe. I'd heard of them, but only because their offices were in one of the most imposing old Georgian buildings in the High Street. I phoned them and made an appointment to see Mr Bentham, their medical negligence specialist, on the 21st of November, the day after I was due to see Professor Shaw in London. It was going to be a busy and traumatic week.

Meanwhile I kept my appointment with Dr Keller, who was a specialist in palliative care. I had to see him at a hospital annexe called 'The Pines'.

"Ah, The Pines," exclaimed my friend Amy when I told her. "A friend of mine with cancer died in there not so long ago – wonderful care."

It dawned on me that The Pines was the local hospice. They *had* written me off. They were preparing me for the end. How was I going to convince this Dr Keller that there was still plenty of life in me, and that the lump and bowel problem could, according to my complimentary therapist, be caused by something other than cancer?

Mike accompanied me to the consultation, and Dr Keller had a trainee with him. He struck me as being rather ill-at-ease, but then a job which entails telling people they are going to die must make any normal person feel uncomfortable. As we went through my medical notes I made it clear that I had doubts about the diagnosis. I suggested the possibility of some kind of infection. I showed him my tongue, which for weeks had had a coating like a furred-up kettle. Didn't doctors look at tongues any more? He didn't seem very interested. He asked about my pain, and seemed rather surprised that it was kept under control with the occasional paracetamol. I was assured that effective pain control would be available when I needed it. He prescribed some kind of foam to squirt up my anus to help with the diarrhoea. I explained that I was seeing Professor Shaw and that I hoped he would investigate my condition more fully. At the end of the consultation, which had lasted nearly an hour, I had the feeling that Dr Keller was as confused about my condition as I was.

The foam was useless. It went everywhere except up my rectum – mostly all over the loo walls. I gave up after three attempts. It was a complete waste of money, along with every other prescribed medicine for my bowels. I was now going so often that I was virtually bowel incontinent.

At 6.45am on the 20th of November Mike and I left home to get to the City and Royal Hospital for my 10am appointment. The plan was to drive to the outskirts of London and then take the tube to the city centre. But we hadn't driven to London for years and we had totally underestimated the density of the morning traffic on the motorway.

"This is a complete waste of time," I complained to Mike. "This prof won't be able to do anything. Let's turn round at the next junction and go home."

"We've come this far, we go on," Mike replied. "You mustn't give up."

When we finally got to the tube station, there was a long wait for a train. I phoned the outpatients' clinic to explain that I'd be about an hour late. Fortunately they seemed neither surprised nor perturbed. I probably wasn't the only country bumpkin referred to them who was totally naïve about London traffic.

We finally got to see Professor Julian Shaw at about 11.30. We were ushered into a small consulting room which rapidly became very crowded. There was me, Mike, a nurse, a student, another doctor, and sitting at the only desk, the Professor. He was grey, balding, and distinguished-looking, more or less how I imagined he would be. He struck me initially as rather brusque in manner, but it was brought on by the fact that here was someone who was totally in control. He had the fortunate knack of oozing confidence without appearing arrogant. I felt in safe hands.

After briefly running through my medical history, and giving me a dire warning that he might not be able to do very much for me, he did a physical examination. There was no separate examination cubicle, the only privacy between the couch and the audience being a flimsy curtain. In some respects the City and Royal was far below the standards of Casterbridge Hospital. He felt my abdomen and then probed up my rectum, causing a lot of discomfort and a slight release of faeces. That seemed to tell him something, and he quickly decided on what further tests I would need.

"I'll need a biopsy," he explained. Surprise, surprise, I

thought. "That will need a general anaesthetic, and while you're under that I'll do a more thorough internal examination which will save you any further pain."

Professor Shaw rose further in my estimation. He appeared kind and considerate, as well as fully in command.

"I'd like to have you in next week," he went on. "We can do the pre-op checks today if you can stay for another hour or two. Are you happy with that?"

"Yes, that's fine." I was pleasantly surprised at how fast things were moving.

He turned to his nurse. "Arrange for Mrs Bland's admission on, er, let's see, the 27th, please."

I was handed over to a junior doctor who dealt with consent forms and other minor details. Then I trailed round various departments having blood tests, a chest X-ray, and an ECG to make sure the old ticker was in order. I hardly had to wait at all. The City and Royal seemed a remarkably efficient hospital, despite the grotty buildings.

"I was very impressed with Prof Shaw," I said to Mike as we sped home down the motorway.

"So was I. He knows what he's doing, and he seems to have a good team. Let's hope he can sort you out. He's certainly not wasting any time, which is a relief."

"It really shows up the poor treatment I was getting at Casterbridge," I observed. "They should have done a biopsy weeks ago. I can't understand why they didn't. It's all confusion and cover-up, I reckon, and a deliberate attempt to write me off."

"It'll be interesting to see what this Mr Bentham makes of it all."

CHAPTER 14

The imposing Georgian mansion housing the offices of Jeffreys and Rowe overlooked a new supermarket and massive car park. The modern development of Casterbridge had been halted just in time to preserve most of the old town, which was now a relatively calm enclave of narrow streets and fine old houses. We bought a pile of toilet rolls and cat food in the supermarket to earn our two hours' free parking, and then kept our appointment with Mr Bentham.

Joseph Bentham appeared to be the stereotypical provincial solicitor – ageing, overweight, and rather tweedy-looking.

I launched into an account of everything that had happened since my operation in February 2000, while he scribbled away furiously on a yellow legal pad.

"Ah, Mr Ellman," he interrupted. "The name is known to me. There have been a number of cases."

That quite encouraged me, and it very much backed up my hairdresser's comment – 'he is not liked'.

I continued, explaining my suspicions that a foreign object had been left in me which had been removed during the September 2000 operation, and that all this had led to a massive cover-up which could now be having an adverse effect on my current care. I brought him right up to date with details of my consultation with Professor Shaw. Then I explained that I had already been through the complaints procedure with the GMC and NHS.

"I'm sorry to say this," he commented, "but you were wasting your time. In my experience no-one has ever got anywhere with the complaints system. You'd have been better coming to me straight away."

"I'd agree. I've just met with whitewash," I replied.

Finally I mentioned the fabricated histology report, the police investigation into it, and my own. Mr Bentham looked doubtful.

"You may have a case against the police, and possibly the GMC, but that seems a side issue."

"But don't you think it's more important than that? It's evidence of wrong-doing at Casterbridge Hospital by someone, almost certainly Ellman. It's the only clear evidence. Everything else is circumstantial."

"But I can't see how it might help with your principal allegation – the botched operation."

"I see it as part of the cover-up, part of the false medical history it seems they've been trying to create."

I was very disappointed at Mr Bentham's attitude towards the fabricated report. Perhaps when he studied events more carefully he would realise how it fitted in and how it could be used. I watched him closely as he perused his scribbled notes. I knew there was a lot for him to absorb.

"I think you do have a case," he stated. "But it's a difficult and complex one. Damages for an unnecessary operation, which is what your case boils down to if indeed the second operation was to correct mistakes made at the first operation, would probably be in the range of five to ten thousand pounds. I wouldn't rate your chances of success as being particularly high. Bearing that in mind, do you wish to proceed?"

"I'm not too interested in the money. I'm mostly interested in finding out what has been going on, and getting my medical notes corrected if there's things in them which are misleading. I'd also like Ellman to be disciplined if he's been acting unprofessionally."

"Yes, I understand your feelings on the matter, but it is my duty as your advisor to make you fully aware of your chances of success, what the case is likely to cost, and what your liabilities might be should your case fail, which, I'm afraid to say, is something you must bear in mind."

"I suppose you mean I'd have to pay the other side's costs if I lost."

"Exactly, so it's not only your own costs which have to be considered." Mr Bentham looked up at Mike and me sitting in front of his desk, and appeared to be studying us closely. "I expect you realise that these days you have to be dirt poor to get legal aid," he said. Was he trying to literally sum us up? We never flaunted our wealth, exotic long-haul holidays being our only extravagance. So, as usual, we were wearing our normal down-market chain store and catalogue clothing, and must have looked as though we had walked off the nearest council estate. Mike was now an old-age pensioner. I was no longer working, largely due to my state of health, but not yet old enough for my pensions to kick in. However, we both had very substantial savings, cutting us out of any kind of means-tested benefits.

"No, we wouldn't get legal aid," I confirmed. "So what sort of costs are we talking about?"

"I'll give you a leaflet about our fee structure, but I should estimate that you must think in terms of at least five thousand pounds even before we can decide whether your case has a good chance of success."

"That's all right," I replied. I knew what professional fees were like. I'd been billing Mike's accountancy clients for years. Already I was mentally doubling the figure mentioned. Basically, at my level of spending, ten thousand pounds represented a new car. I wouldn't need a new car for many years, as my present four-year-old one was completely reliable. To update it would be sheer extravagance, and getting my health problems in order was far more important than getting a shiny new lump of metal in the garage. If I won my case, the other side would pay my legal expenses and whatever damages I was awarded. It was a bit of a gamble, but one worth taking if only for peace of mind.

"Now, we must think about time scales," Mr Bentham went on. "When did you say the first operation took place?"

"The 1st of February 2000."

"Oh dear. The problem is there's a three year time limit for bringing your sort of action, which means we have only, let's see, less than ten weeks to issue a summons. That's cutting things very fine, especially with Christmas intervening."

"I did know about the three year limit," I told him, "but I thought I'd left plenty of time."

Mr Bentham smiled ruefully. "Never mind. We'll just have to get moving. I'm going to need a full statement from you. Do you keep a diary?"

"Yes. I jot down what I do every day."

"Good. You must include in your statement the dates of all consultations, examinations, operations, and so forth. If you can do it on a computer and let us have the disc, it will be easier for us this end to make any necessary alterations. Can you do that?"

"No problem. I'll try and get it done before I go up to the City and Royal next Wednesday."

"I'll also need all your medical notes."

"I've got them from January 2000 to February 2001. Do you want copies?"

"It's better if I get them from source myself. I'll need all your records from Casterbridge, the City and Royal, and from your GP."

"You won't get anything before 1995 from Casterbridge because they told me the records prior to then have been destroyed." Mr Bentham looked rather surprised.

"I think you'll find that although the actual paper records might have been destroyed, they will almost certainly have been transferred to microfiche," he explained in his rather pedantic way.

I was fast reaching the conclusion that Mr Bentham had a serious case of verbal diarrhoea. He would always use twenty words where one would do, so lengthening his consultations and therefore racking up his fee. However, to be fair, I was so ignorant about aspects of the law that some points had to be carefully explained to me, and he did this well.

"We must get moving," he said once more. "Let's hope this leads to a successful case. Mr Ellman has already escaped being struck off by the skin of his teeth. Doctors like him shouldn't be allowed to continue in practice. He's a disgrace to his profession. Most doctors are competent, decent, and hard-working. The profession can do without people like Ellman."

The almost unprofessional vehemence of these remarks took me by surprise. Mr Bentham obviously knew far more about the devious ways of Ellman than I ever would. It was almost as if he was pursuing some kind of personal vendetta. Anyway, it seemed I had found the right man to conduct my case.

During the following days I spent hours at Mike's computer compiling my statement. What with the unfamiliar technology, having to refer to my diaries, and drag unpleasant details from my memory, it was a very tiring task. My bowels were really bad, which made it difficult to concentrate. Whatever damages I might get, I felt I was earning them. Mr Bentham had also requested details of the nature and outcome of my GMC and NHS complaints, so I had to go through all that correspondence as well. Despite condensing things as much as I could, the statement still stretched to nine sides of closely printed A4.

On the 27th of November I travelled up to the City and Royal, feeling satisfied that I had now got my legal case up and running. It was now over to Mr Bentham. I felt reasonably confident that Casterbridge Hospital would quickly agree to an out-of-court settlement once they had received details of my claim from the County Court. But whether I would ever learn the full details of what had been going on was another matter. It had been explained to me that my case had to be against Casterbridge Hospital, as Ellman was an employee. I rather hoped he would not be employed there for much longer. It seemed that he had already blotted his copybook. He had probably been going along like a driver with nine penalty points on his licence. One more strike and he'd be out. Quite possibly it was this thought that had driven him to embark on such an elaborate cover-up when he realised he had botched things yet again.

I had recognised from early on that a weakness in my scenario was that the obvious way for a surgeon to proceed when a foreign object had been left in a patient would be to admit the mistake immediately. I would have had another operation before the incision had started healing, and would have received a small sum in compensation along with apologies and assurances that operating procedures were to be reviewed, or some such rubbish. Ellman might have been subjected to some minor disciplinary measures if it was thought he was to blame in any way. It would all have been quite simple and reasonably satisfactory. The fact that there had been previous cases against Ellman now meant I could dismiss the niggling doubt about a possible weakness in my case. I became increasingly confident of a successful outcome.

I thought about everything as the National Express coach sped along the motorway. Coach travel was slower and cheaper than rail, but the principal advantage was that all passengers had to be seated. I could not risk having to stand in my enfeebled condition. All the coaches had on-board loos, and I had seated myself conveniently close to it for my frequent visits.

I arrived at the City and Royal in the early afternoon, but

had to wait three hours before a bed became available. A junior doctor came and explained what was to be done under anaesthetic. It involved passing a needle up my vagina and taking a sample of tissue from the lump, the needle being guided by X-ray. It all sounded quite clever and not too invasive. Why hadn't it been done at Casterbridge Hospital? At the same time Professor Shaw would have a good poke around up my various orifices without causing me any pain. I was then asked if I had any questions.

"Yes," I said, finding that for once my mind hadn't gone a blank at this point. "Assuming this lump is largely fluid-filled, won't it be like puncturing a water-filled balloon?"

"Not really. Any fluid there will be in small sacks, so at worst we would only expect a small release of fluid."

"Well, I suppose you know what you're doing," I replied doubtfully. "So how long will I be in for?"

"If you lived close by you'd be able to go home tomorrow evening, but as you have a long journey I think it would be best if you wait until Friday afternoon, just to be sure everything is OK. Can someone come and take you home?"

"My husband will have to come up and travel back with me."

The following morning I was taken to the theatre for what was called a guided needle biopsy. When I came round in the recovery room and asked the time, I realised I had been unconscious for about one and a half hours, whereas I had expected to be out for about half an hour at most. I also had a catheter inserted which I had not expected. Once more it appeared things had not gone to plan. Someone told me that something more than just a biopsy had been done and that the doctors would explain what had happened. I was taken back to the ward and then transferred to another. What the hell was going on? Then I was put on an antibiotic intravenous drip. That strongly suggested infection of some kind. Perhaps Terry Sutton had been right.

At last a junior doctor appeared.

"We found quite a lot of pus and fluid," she explained. "We drained it off, so the lump should have gone down."

She pulled back the bed covers and gently felt my abdomen. "Yes, that's much better. There's not much there now. You'll need this antibiotic for a few days," she said, indicating the drip, "so I'm afraid you won't be going home tomorrow."

"So when will I be going home?"

"About the middle of next week I would guess. We did manage to get a biopsy, and I think Prof wants the results of the lab analysis so he can discuss it with you before you go home."

As the little entourage accompanying her moved on, I heard the words 'pelvic abscess' mentioned. So, what Casterbridge had diagnosed as extensive, incurable cancer was, in fact, massive infection. It was beyond belief. What would have happened if the abscess had burst? I would have died unless I had got very prompt and appropriate treatment. Events now suggested strongly that the results of the CT scan had been deliberately misinterpreted so that they fitted better with the ultrasound scan results of August 2000. I had seen that report among my notes, and it mentioned some kind of structure consisting of many small cells, rather like a sponge, in fact, surprise, surprise. But it seemed that the mass now in me had probably been more like a cyst, and I was more convinced than ever that it was something new that had started forming in the spring when I first started getting bowel problems. Now the cover-up was indeed compromising my care. All I could hope was that now I was in a different hospital under a new consultant, matters could be totally reviewed. But would that be done if it meant revealing the extent of the cover-up? I doubted it. To what extent was Professor Shaw his own man? A lot would depend on that.

Despite everything, I had to accept that something was seriously wrong in my pelvis. What was causing these cysts and abscesses? I had to take on board the possibility that they could be related to underlying cancer. How long would I have to wait for the biopsy results?

I phoned Mike and explained everything to him. He had already bought the coach tickets to come up and escort me home the next day, but instead he came laden with odds and ends to keep me comfortable and reasonably happy in a ward which seemed to specialise in sensory deprivation. There wasn't even bedside radio, and the TV in the day room had terrible reception and always seemed to be tuned to the soaps which, it seemed, was all my fellow patients wanted to watch. Although the standard of the medical staff and the general organisation seemed far superior to Casterbridge, the actual physical condition of the wards left much to be desired.

The following day turned out to be rather confusing and miserable. The catheter was uncomfortable, my bowels were as bad as ever, and now I had a discharge from my vagina, which I was told was likely to last for a few days as remaining fluid drained off. The doctors were quite openly speaking of infection, and I had more antibiotic drips. My treatment plan seemed unclear, but it appeared I would be kept in until either a CT or MRI scan could be done, and until the biopsy results were available.

Mike arrived just before 1pm after a four hour door-to-door journey. It wasn't officially visiting hours but nobody minded when they realised how far he had travelled. He stayed just over an hour, much of which was taken up with me instructing him to cancel various appointments and social arrangements to accommodate my unexpected stay in hospital. I thought how old and tired Mike looked. After all, he was nearly sixty-seven, ten years older than me. He would have found the journey very trying.

"Don't come up again until I'm ready to be taken home," I instructed him. "It's just ridiculous – eight hours travel for an hour or so here. We can talk on the phone every evening, and if I desperately need something, you could post it."

He sat there for a while, no doubt taking in the grotty condition of the ward and the multi-racial nature of both the staff and patients. It was like the United Nations in the City and Royal, and everyone seemed to get on very well. A black lady in the bed opposite sat reading her bible, while a few beds along an Asian lady lay propped up in bed with a voluminous headscarf draped round her head and shoulders. Meanwhile the mainly Filipino and Zimbabwean nurses went about their duties.

"So what do you think about developments?" I asked Mike.

"I'm not entirely surprised. Perhaps matters will now be clarified."

"Perhaps, or perhaps not. Not if it means revealing the cover-up that's been going on. You'd better let Bentham know about things."

"You've got to get it into your head that no one's going to spill the beans to you, even if they do understand what's probably been going on. All the same, I think Shaw will do his best for you."

"And be economical with the truth?"

"No doubt, and don't you go stirring things."

With that sound advice Mike prepared to go. He'd brought me some books, audio tapes, a small radio/cassette player, extra pyjamas, and my little Psion organiser on which I could play chess, Scrabble, and patience. I was quite good at amusing myself, which was fortunate seeing I wouldn't be getting any more visits.

The following day, a Saturday, the catheter was removed, and I had the last antibiotic drip. Free of bags and leads, I could now move around more easily. I began to feel better, which was probably due to the antibiotics dealing with the infection. However, the increased activity aggravated the vaginal discharge, although whatever it was coming out was better out than in.

Early in the evening I phoned Mike. There had been a letter from Bentham. Mike had opened it and gave me the gist of it. It seemed that as time was so short, he was already seeking advice from counsel, by which he meant a barrister, as to how he should proceed. He had instructed a Jeremy Carr on all matters – the possible medical negligence, the forged medical documents, the inadequate police enquiry, and the unsatisfactory GMC investigation. He was being very thorough, and I was glad he was taking the forgery issue seriously.

After the phone call, a boring evening stretched ahead of me. There was only one thing to do – go to bed with a good book. I settled back on the pillows and propped up 'Down Under' by Bill Bryson on my raised knees. Soon I was dreaming of a holiday in Australia, health permitting. We could rent a car and tour, drive through the desert to Ayres Rock, see koala bears, go to the Sydney Opera House....

"Mrs Bland?"

I looked up. Professor Julian Shaw was standing at the end of my bed holding my file. What on earth was a very top consultant doing in an NHS ward at seven o'clock on a Saturday night? Surely he'd done his share of unsocial hours as a junior doctor, and now he'd expect his own minions to provide cover except in dire emergencies, and I was hardly in that category.

"Oh! Hello, Professor Shaw."

"I thought I'd better explain to you what happened the other day. We drained about a litre of mucus-like fluid from your pelvis, and you've probably lost a little more since then."

"Yes, quite a lot."

"We've got to find out what's causing it to form, so I'd like you to stay here for an MRI scan, hopefully on Tuesday. You should be feeling a lot better now."

"Yes, I am."

"Good. Your bowel function should also improve. It's a good job we didn't open you up." He sort of rolled his eyes heavenwards, the implication being, I think, that it could have been extremely messy, and that they'd still be steam-cleaning the theatre ceiling. "I'm going to have to reassess your case," he continued, "but things are looking much better for you."

He moved forward and placed a reassuring hand on my knee raised under the covers. He was dressed smartly but casually in an open-neck check shirt and a leather blouson.

"Thank you for letting me know," I said.

He looked down at me. I had the feeling he wanted to say more. But then he was gone. It seemed he'd just come to see me. He certainly wasn't on a regular ward round, and his registrar was minding the fort that night. So had he just dropped in on his way to some fashionable dinner party in Islington or somewhere? Isn't that what top consultants did on Saturday nights if they hadn't retreated to their yachts or country cottages? And why had he been alone? All the other consultants visiting their patients seemed to go around with enormous gangs. The least surprising thing was the news he had given me.

I went to the ward phone again and got Mike.

"You'll never guess! I've just seen Prof Shaw – on a Saturday night! He says he's going to reassess my case, but that things look much better for me."

"That's good. I think we're getting somewhere."

"D'you know what I reckon? I reckon the CT scan report from Casterbridge was faked in some way. Surely otherwise it would have shown a big fluid-filled mass."

"It all seems very suspicious," Mike conceded. "Anyway, it seems Shaw is dealing with things in his own way."

I went back to bed, but I didn't read much. Although everything was looking up, it was all becoming very complicated. If he wasn't careful Shaw would find himself dragged into the cover-up. I didn't want that. I'd have to tell him that I was taking legal action against Casterbridge Hospital. That should focus his mind. But how and when should I do it?

That night I wrote in my diary 'It could be a massive case'.

CHAPTER 15

I had to wait until the following Thursday for a scan, and then it was a CT scan, not an MRI, but I was assured it was just as good for determining the nature of the tumour. The result of the biopsy still hadn't come through when Mike came up to escort me home on the following day, but I was told I would be informed by phone of the result and the scan findings as soon as they were available.

With the unexpectedly long stay in hospital (nine days instead of two) there was a lot of catching-up to do. I gave top priority to an additional statement for Bentham about the unexpected events at the City and Royal. In my covering letter I emphasised the mental torture inflicted on me by the doctors at Casterbridge Hospital. Had a biopsy been carried out much sooner, the pelvic abscess would have been discovered and treated, saving me weeks of pain. I pointed out that recent events had virtually proved that a cover-up had been going on, and that it seemed there had been a deliberate attempt to deny me necessary treatment in the hope that I would die. Understandably, I now had a deep suspicion of all doctors.

On the 11th of December I had the promised phone call from the City and Royal. The biopsy had not revealed any obvious cancer, only the borderline changes which had been present back at the time of the February 2000 operation. The CT scan showed that the lump had gone down, but that there was still fluid present which would have to be removed once it had been decided how best to do it. It all seemed quite good news. Cancer now seemed a remote possibility although I knew it couldn't be completely ruled out. I had an out-patient appointment with Professor Shaw for the following week when we'd be able to discuss matters more fully.

I had almost forgotten about the letter I had sent to the Royal College of Pathologists on the 9th of October about the fact that Dr Appleyard could not have been a consultant by 1981 if he had qualified in 1977. Then, on the 16th of December, I received a reply. It was the most appalling whitewash I had ever read. It started quite well by acknowledging that Appleyard could not have been a consultant in 1981, but then it said it had been the practice in the past for trainee pathologists to sign their own investigations, albeit under the supervision of a consultant. However, I reasoned, that would not entitle them to describe themselves as a consultant. That fact, it seemed, had been completely overlooked. The letter then went off at a tangent, going into great detail about how, in the 1980s, initial histopathology reports were handwritten, and then typed, with the handwritten reports remaining filed in the laboratory. It was all the usual obfuscation by irrelevant detail which I was now quite used to. As I now knew that not only was Appleyard not a consultant in 1981 but also that he was not working at Casterbridge Hospital at that time, everything struck me as a fanciful concoction put together by top people at the Royal College of Pathologists who should have known better. It also made me suspect even more strongly that the police had never consulted Appleyard. Had they done so, he would have pointed out to them that he was not a consultant in 1981, and would not have described himself as one. I decided to send a copy of the letter to the solicitor.

On the 18th of December I travelled to the City and Royal once more for an out-patient appointment with Professor Shaw. I was expecting things to be quite straightforward. I would tell him that I was feeling much better, although still suffering from frequent bowel movements, and he would have decided upon what further needed doing. Instead it turned out to be one of the most confusing consultations I had ever had. It began badly when I pointed out that there appeared to be an error on my discharge form made out when I left the hospital. The terms used to describe my cancer had been switched round so that it appeared that the obvious cancer found in 1981 had been found after the February 2000 operation, and that the borderline condition had been found in 1981. This may well have been a quite genuine and fully understandable mistake seeing that cancer progresses from borderline to a more advanced form over time. However, I couldn't help being suspicious. Were the City and Royal now perpetuating the deliberate misinterpretation of my condition at Casterbridge? Would I ever be free of this terrible muddle?

"I think the diagnoses have been switched round," I tried to explain. "I had the full-blown cancer in 1981. It was only borderline in 2000."

"Professor Shaw looked at the copy of the discharge form in my file.

"This is correct," he said.

"I don't think it is. The terms should be the other way round. I didn't have cancer in 2000, just some borderline changes."

"The terms used are correct," Professor Shaw insisted. Because I didn't fully understand the histological terminology it was impossible to argue with him, but I knew I was correct. All I could hope for was that Shaw would realise this when, or if, he looked more closely at my notes.

"Now, at the operation in 1998..." he went on.

"You mean 2000."

He adjusted his glasses and appeared to be reading something in my file. "In 1998..."

"Perhaps you mean 1981," I said with some exasperation.

"I didn't have any contact with Casterbridge Hospital in 1998. I had my first op in 1981, the second in February 2000, and the third in September 2000. Nothing happened in 1998."

Professor Shaw looked totally confused. I began to wonder whether it was actually my file he had in front of him, or was he reading some complete bilge sent from Casterbridge in which they had constructed a false medical history to support what now appeared to be an erroneous cancer diagnosis? This was terrible. I had placed great faith and trust in Professor Shaw, but now he seemed to have totally lost the plot. Was he genuinely confused, or had he been corrupted by the scheming doctors at Casterbridge?

He stopped looking at my notes and looked up at me.

"Anyway, how are you feeling now?" he asked.

"I'm feeling much better now, thank you. I've still got a slight vaginal discharge. The bowels are a bit better, but not right."

"The discharge will stop in time, but I don't expect the bowels to get any better. You see, the CT scan shows there is still a mass pressing on your rectum. It's smaller since the release of all that fluid, but it's not going to go away. May I examine you again?"

"Of course."

This time I was in a consulting room with a separate examination cubicle. Sally, his nurse, got me ready on the couch and then Shaw appeared, pulled on latex gloves, smeared a finger with jelly, and delved painfully into my intimate orifices. That seemed to tell him quite a lot.

"It's as I thought. The mass is low down between the vagina and rectum. If it's removed surgically it would mean taking out a section of your rectum and that would probably mean a permanent colostomy."

"I'm not having that," I said decisively as I sat up on the couch. I'd seen a drawing of a colostomy bag in my medical encyclopedia, and there was no way I wanted to live the rest of my life with a bag of shit stuck to my tum. It was difficult to think of anything worse.

"Well, you see," Professor Shaw explained, "there's very little to play with so low down on the bowel, so it's unlikely the bowel could be joined up again. But I can understand your concerns, so we'll consider alternatives."

I went back to the consulting room, where a Dr Galton had joined us. It was explained that he was an oncologist who worked alongside Shaw as the chemotherapy expert.

"I trained Dr Oswald," he said. And he didn't do a very good job, I thought to myself. He was hardly likely to doubt Oswald's diagnosis of incurable cancer, so it seemed that although Shaw had not found obvious signs of cancer, the cancer threat was still very much present.

"We could try a short course of chemotherapy," Dr Galton said. "You could have it at Casterbridge under Dr Oswald."

That suggestion horrified me. I didn't want any more to do with Oswald or Casterbridge Hospital, but neither did I want to travel all the way to the City and Royal for chemotherapy. I got the feeling that Shaw and his team were rather anxious to get rid of me. Perhaps they could sense trouble.

"It doesn't seem a good idea to have an unpleasant and potentially harmful treatment for a disease I might not even have," I said.

Dr Galton seemed to take that on board. "That is a point. And the chances of chemotherapy being effective for your borderline condition is quite low."

"I'd also like to wait and see what is happening about the Octeotride treatment Dr Oswald mentioned. I still haven't heard if my cells are compatible, or whatever."

Galton and Shaw looked at each other, but said nothing. Surely they would know of the drug and have their own views about it. The atmosphere seemed strange.

I have to go now," Dr Galton said, glancing at his watch. "I hope all goes well for you."

I remained in the room with Professor Shaw and his nurse.

I think the best thing to do at the moment is to closely monitor your condition," Professor Shaw concluded. "We'll have another MRI scan."

"How can I have *another* MRI scan when I've never had one?" I exploded.

"You've never had an MRI scan?" Professor Shaw said, raising his eyebrows in surprise.

"No. Only ultrasound and CT scans."

Sally, looking equally surprised, spoke up. "So you've never been in the tube-like machine that makes the funny noises?"

"Never."

"Well, I think you'd remember it if you had been, as it's not very pleasant," Sally added. She exchanged what I interpreted as a meaningful glance with Professor Shaw. Now I was more certain than ever that Casterbridge Hospital had sent the City and Royal a pack of lies. Should I now tell Professor Shaw that I had commenced legal action against Casterbridge Hospital? If he wasn't careful, he would be drawn into the mess, and I didn't want that.

"Book Mrs Bland for an MRI scan," Professor Shaw instructed Sally. He turned to me. "I have to go now, but I'll see you again in a few weeks to discuss the MRI scan." He left me with an anxious-looking Sally.

"I'm so confused," I said, feeling close to tears.

"Professor Shaw is confused too," Sally confided. "There seem to be gaps in your records from Casterbridge."

I thought quickly. This was probably because there were no clinical reports to back up fake information given in some covering letter. I got the impression that after his unexpected findings during the biopsy, Professor Shaw had investigated my case more thoroughly than anyone would have expected. He himself would now be highly suspicious, but he would never let on to me. Perhaps some of the things he had said had been quite deliberate to assess my reactions, which then possibly confirmed his own suspicions.

"If there's a difference between what comes from Casterbridge and what I say, you must believe me," I said.

"Yes, we'll do that," Sally assured me.

"You see, I don't trust them at Casterbridge. After the September 2000 operation I was told the lump was reactive swelling which would go down naturally." I wondered whether I should voice my opinions about a foreign object, but decided to leave it at that. I didn't want to appear a paranoid nutcase.

Sally filled in a form for an MRI scan some time in January, and I left. It was a lovely winter's day and as I had some time to kill before the coach went, I walked westwards along the Embankment towards Victoria Coach Station. The journey took over an hour, and although I was a little footsore towards the end, I concluded there couldn't be too much wrong with me.

Everything that had happened at the consultation was reported to Mr Bentham, as I felt it all helped my case. We were now engaged in frequent correspondence, and it quickly became obvious that Bentham was as verbose in his letters as he was in conversation. However, he did seem to be moving as fast as was possible in the legal profession. He was most concerned about the time limitation issue, and because my first contact with Ellman's team had been on the 10th of January 2000, he thought it best to have the summons in court just before that date in 2003 to be within the three year time limit. Fortunately an outline summons could be issued without the case being fully prepared. There was then a four-month period in which all the evidence could be prepared. Even this could be extended if good reason could be shown. Bentham had evidently concluded that I had a good case because there was a court fee of £500 to issue the summons. I rather hoped he would not put me to that expense if he thought my case was frivolous. He was now busy obtaining my notes from Casterbridge Hospital, the City and Royal, and my GP. Counsel, Jeremy Carr, had been instructed to give initial advice on how to proceed, and a top gynaecologist was being lined up to give an expert opinion once my notes were available. Thought would be given as to whether a report from a bowel specialist would be necessary, and whether a psychiatrist should assess the psychological trauma I had suffered.

I provided further evidence in the form of photocopies of relevant diary entries, and I also sent Bentham a copy of the tape of the consultation with Mr Harcourt. I explained that I had taken this rather sneaky action because of the trouble I had had about who said what at a previous consultation with Ellman. I made it clear that I was not in the habit of secretly taping my consultations. I also provided a cheque for £2,200 for the work done to date, and I knew I would now be writing cheques for similar amounts for some time. However, I was convinced that it would all pay off in the end.

CHAPTER 16

Christmas 2002 came and went with me hardly noticing it. I was too wrapped up in my medical problems and my fast-moving legal action. At the end of the year I spent some time looking at old diaries, and generally thinking about everything. The medics appeared to hold the view that I had had cancer ever since 1981, and that it had been slowly developing. Yet in 1987 I had been proclaimed cured by Dr Carson. I had had no treatment for cancer since the radiotherapy in 1981, and no symptoms until December 1999. If what I had now was indeed cancer, surely it should be considered a new episode rather than a late recurrence. I didn't understand the time scales doctors used, although I did vaguely have it in my head that one was considered cured if there was no recurrence within five years of the original diagnosis. Then it was unlikely that cancer would recur, which, presumably, was why my check-ups ended five and a half years after the 1981 diagnosis.

I had the feeling that Casterbridge Hospital had given Professor Shaw the impression that I had had on-going cancer for many years. The whole cancer issue had been blown out of all proportion as part of the grand cover-up. While I couldn't afford to totally dismiss the possibility of cancer, the advanced and incurable disease diagnosed by Oswald was clearly utter tosh. The fact that Shaw had detected what he termed gaps in my records from Casterbridge did indeed suggest that dates had been glossed over to give the impression that what had happened in 1981 had gone on in 1998. But why 1998? Perhaps that was because the days of the week (Monday, Tuesday etc) had the same dates in 1981 as they did in 1998. It's amazing what looking at old diaries will reveal. If dates of tests and examinations were somehow being shifted from 1981 to 1998 there would be no chance of the embarrassment of them occurring on a weekend. Well, that was one possible explanation. Another was that a first occurrence of cancer in 1998 might fit in with what would appear to be a natural progression of the disease. It was all very confusing and very worrying, and I really didn't know what to do about it. I certainly didn't want to alienate Shaw because I felt he was my only chance of getting effective treatment. Despite his nurse, Sally, assuring me that they would believe my version of events, I still suspected that he might believe the fairy tales from Casterbridge Hospital. But surely he would ask himself why the patient was producing a different version of events. Would he put it down to some sort of mental aberration caused by the stress of the cancer diagnosis? There's nothing worse than being considered mad when you're not.

Events soon got going in the new year. Bentham wrote to say he was slowly getting all my medical notes together. He was already referring to the case as 'complex'. He had decided that the notes had to be paginated and indexed by a special company. More expense, I thought, but almost certainly a necessary one. I think Bentham was already cautiously optimistic that I had a good case, and that there would be a very good pay-out in professional fees for him and his cronies as well as damages for me. The big problem for me was how much I was going to have to spend before I knew for sure I would win. Instinct told me that £10,000 should be my upper limit. I could lose that without noticing it too much, but I would have to be prepared to abandon my case if things were still unclear at that point. The other possibility was a no win, no fee agreement, what the legal profession calls a conditional fee agreement (CFA). The client doesn't pay anything up front, but if the case is won all the fees due are doubled and then paid by the losing side. For understandable reasons these agreements are only entered into if there appears a better than fifty-fifty chance of winning. It was still too soon to judge accurately whether I would succeed, so there was no point in asking for a CFA at this stage.

On the 8th of January I received an appointment to see Dr Oswald again. I had not expected it, as I thought I was now totally under the care of Shaw at the City and Royal. I phoned his secretary to cancel it, explaining that I wanted Shaw to deal with my case now. I didn't add that I had no intention of seeking treatment at a hospital I was about to sue. The secretary said that it was Shaw who had requested that I saw Oswald again. So what was Shaw's game? Hadn't he recognised the fact that I was disillusioned and deeply suspicious about my treatment at Casterbridge Hospital? Was he trying to get rid of me because he smelt big trouble?

On the 10th of January I received a phone call from Natalie Yeo, the Macmillan nurse at Casterbridge. She asked how I was. I detected a strange hesitancy in her voice, as if she had been told to contact me, but didn't really want to do so. Sometimes the phone brings out nuances in the voice which are not noticed during face-to-face conversations. If she had been attached to a lie-detecting machine, I felt it would be going haywire.

I replied in polite but slightly sarcastic tones.

"I'm feeling much better, thank you. What Dr Oswald had told me was incurable cancer turned out to be largely a pelvic abscess. It was drained at the City and Royal and my pain has gone. But my bowels still aren't right. They think there's still something there, so I'm having an MRI scan on the 14th. Then Professor Shaw will decide what to do."

"Oh, I see." She sounded surprised at my news, but I got the feeling she already knew what had happened.

"There's no point in seeing Dr Oswald again until we have the MRI scan results," I went on.

"Would you like me to cancel the appointment?"

"I've already done that." I paused, wondering whether I could push her into revealing what she might know, or rather what she might be prepared to tell me. I knew that deep down she was a very caring and honest person, but that she was caught in an awkward situation. "Er, this abscess, it came as a bit of a surprise. What do you think caused it?"

"I really couldn't say. Anyway, I'm glad you're feeling a bit better. I hope your scan goes OK."

She couldn't get off the line fast enough. I knew I had touched on a sensitive area. I had already asked the doctors at the City and Royal about the causes of pelvic abscesses. Diverticular disease was one possible explanation, but so was infection following pelvic operations. Any good nurse would know that and would have mentioned it. If any foreign objects had indeed been left in me, they might not all have been removed during the September 2000 operation. A small fragment of a swab or sponge could then become the focus for infection. I had the feeling that Natalie knew exactly what had been going on. Had her superiors forced her into some kind of fishing expedition to try and judge what I myself might know or suspect? Were they worried about what their colleagues at the City and Royal might have told me? It gave me a certain satisfaction to think that a few doctors at Casterbridge might be shitting themselves nearly as much as I was.

The phone call was reported to Bentham. He had asked me to inform him of all developments in what was very much an on-going and constantly changing case. It was up to him to decide what might be significant and useful.

I had an MRI scan at the City and Royal on 14th January. Sally was right – it wasn't particularly pleasant. I was strapped to a hard narrow stretcher and slid into something that looked like a sewage pipe. Then for about an hour I was subjected to curious noises like someone banging on the outside of the pipe. The foam earplugs I had been given were not very effective. I lay there feeling grateful that I didn't suffer from claustrophobia, and trying to doze, without much success.

Meanwhile Bentham had been busy. A claim against Casterbridge Hospital NHS Trust had been registered in Casterbridge County Court, and we now had four months to collect together notes, obtain a report from an independent gynaecologist, have a conference with Jeremy Carr, the barrister, and present the particulars of the claim. Bentham had already obtained my GP's notes, copies of which he sent me. They dated back to 1951 when I had had whooping cough at the age of five, just after I'd started school. I paid little attention to anything prior to December 1999 which had been when my present troubles had begun. From that point I went through everything very carefully, checking every entry, and every letter and report from the hospital which had found its way into my GP's notes. As well as checking accuracy, I had to be alert to possible omissions. If there had been anything incriminating in the file, the chances are that it would have been removed before the file was copied. It was something that would be very difficult to detect.

As I worked my way through, everything appeared to be in order. Then I came across two letters written by Ellman to Dr Foyle in March 2001, which would have been the time I was complaining to the GMC about my suspicions. The first letter, dated the 23rd of March, mentioned my complaint to the GMC, emphasised that I needed on-going management, but concluded – 'it will not be in any way possible for me to continue seeing her and I am afraid that she will have to explore alternative arrangements. I will try and communicate with you by phone regarding this'. It was quite clear that Ellman expected Foyle to deal with the matter, presumably by contacting me to discuss the situation. If it had been up to

142

me to take the initiative in the matter, Ellman would have written to me, not the GP.

The second letter, dated 28th March, mentioned that I had failed to attend an appointment with him, which had not surprised him in the circumstances. He wanted me to seek care elsewhere, and concluded – 'May I therefore leave it up to you to rearrange'. It was crystal-clear that he had wiped his hands of me. At that point my care had reverted back to Dr Foyle, and if he had heeded Ellman's advice, he could have arranged for my care under a new consultant. Why hadn't he done that? Why hadn't he contacted me to try and sort things out?

I looked at the copies of the GP's handwritten file notes to see what action, if any, had been taken at the time he would have received the letters. On 6th April someone had written 'see letters from Mr Ellman'. That was all. So what about the phone call Ellman had mentioned in the first letter? Was it ever made? If so, the contents should have been noted in my file. Had Dr Foyle made any attempt to phone Ellman? Questions, questions! It slowly dawned on me what had probably happened. There must have been a strictly off-the-record phone call, with Ellman reminding Foyle about the botched operation and subsequent cover-up, which I felt sure Foyle had already been told about. Then it must have gone on:

Ellman: "Looks like the bitch has rumbled me."

Foyle: "Well, you didn't listen. I told you she wasn't born yesterday. Her husband's pretty switched on as well."

Ellman: "So what do you think she'll do now, other than whine to the GMC about me?"

Foyle: "Nothing. I reckon she thinks she's perfectly well. She's not been in here since, er, last May,"

Ellman: "She's probably right. Let's hope she is OK. We're into a nightmare scenario if she isn't."

Foyle: "But I think I'm right in saying there's some question mark over the cancer aspect. She should be having regular monitoring."

Ellman: "Strictly speaking, yes."

Foyle: "So really I should refer her to a new consultant, shouldn't I?"

Ellman: "But that means dragging someone else into the, er, picture. Who? Any suggestions?

Foyle: (Big sigh) "This gets worse and worse. You're expecting me to put your interests before those of my patient."

Ellman: "Of course. I know you will. You owe me – remember that 'premature menopause' case? You'd be struck off if I hadn't kept my mouth shut."

Foyle: "OK, OK. But I suppose you realise I could be in the shit as well as you if it all comes out. It's one thing to keep one's mouth shut, but quite another to, er, actively connive."

Ellman: "Doing nothing is hardly being active. Busy GPs forget things, don't they?

Foyle: "Not cases of ovarian cancer. D'you know, I've only seen one other case in my whole career. No, I won't forget Mrs Bland in a hurry."

Ellman: "That makes two of us."

Foyle: "So what do you want me to do if she comes in demanding referral to a new consultant?"

Ellman: "Get back to me. If the worst comes to the worst, there's someone at Titchmouth...."

I could imagine Dr Foyle banging down the phone, knowing he was caught between the devil and the deep blue sea. Doctors close ranks. They always have, and probably always will. But although they would never whistle-blow on each other, except in extreme cases such as Shipman, most will do their best to avoid being dragged into messes created by colleagues. By not referring me to a new consultant, and not impressing upon me the importance of further check-ups, Foyle had been in breach of his duty of care to me. It surprised me that a doctor who had treated me well for nearly twenty years could do such a thing. Who could you trust?

I wondered whether my legal action should now be widened to include Foyle. It would complicate matters considerably. Ellman was still the main culprit. Foyle had just been dragged into it, no doubt much against his will. Possibly Ellman did have some kind of hold over him, but that was only my fertile imagination. Perhaps doctors were indeed willing to risk their own careers to protect colleagues. It was up to Bentham and Carr to decide what to do. I noted Foyle's negligent non-action along with a few other relatively minor discrepancies which I had noticed in my file.

I moved on to more recent events. There were copies of letters written by the hospital consultants I had seen over the last few months. I had not seen these before because Bentham had not yet obtained the more recent notes from Casterbridge Hospital. One letter was the referral from Harcourt to Oswald. Parts of it were very inaccurate. It said I had had two laparotomies within three years, when, in fact, the two 2000 operations had been seven months apart. I wondered if it had been a deliberate error to imply that there had been a longer time period in which the mysterious lump could develop. There was also a copy of the referral letter Oswald had written to Professor Shaw. That was accurate regarding dates, but I wondered whether Shaw had been looking at Harcourt's letter when he mentioned the year 1998. The phrase 'within three years' implied that my two operations had been between two and three years apart, so if the second operation was in September 2000, the first would have been some time before September 1998. It seemed a feasible explanation for Shaw's strange error.

All this was added to my observations for Bentham. To me it seemed to be evidence that Harcourt and Oswald had been dragged into the conspiracy by Ellman, and that between them they had cooked up some subtle variations on the truth to convey a case of slowly developing, on-going ovarian cancer. No wonder Shaw's nurse had mentioned their confusion. I suspected that Shaw was not yet aware of the facts, but that he soon would be, one way or another. All I could hope was that it wouldn't compromise my care.

Soon after I had dealt with the GP's notes, Bentham sent copies of notes from Casterbridge Hospital. I had to go through these page by page, not only to check accuracy, but to detect whether anything incriminating might have been removed. I was able to check most of them against the notes I had already received when dealing with my earlier complaint to the GMC. It was only the stuff since September 2002 which was new, and some of that I had already seen in the GP's notes.

Within a few minutes I was jotting down some suspicious and possibly significant findings. I was comparing the earlier notes with the copies I had received in March 2001. Reading through Ellman's handwritten notes on our ill-tempered consultation on the 6th of November 2000, I noticed that the latest notes had a written-on addition, something that looked like 'aBH=borderline'. It seemed to be information which would suggest the existence of borderline cancer. Why had it not been written at the time of the consultation? There is bound to be suspicion when a doctor alters, or adds to his notes at a later date. Shipman did that to suggest that some of his victims had heart problems. It was a finding which appeared to support my tentative idea that the cancer aspect was now being talked up as part of the cover-up. Then I noticed an omission. The earlier notes contained a sheet with information about the multi-disciplinary meeting; it was missing from the recent bundle. I had always doubted whether the meeting had actually taken place, and my initial reaction was that reference to it had been removed because my doubts were accurate. It was fortunate that I had obtained my notes in 2001, because otherwise these additions and subtractions would have been undetectable.

What else was missing, I wondered? In 2001 I had only

received notes dating back to 2000. Now I had stuff from 1981 onwards as well, despite the fact that I had previously been told that these had been destroyed. Somewhere there should be the original 1981 histology report from which the forgery had been constructed. Although I found the diagnosis typed out on to another form produced at that time, there appeared to be no original pathology lab report, and therefore no sign of Dr Appleyard's name or signature. It therefore seemed that Ellman really had just picked a likely name to give the fake report the appearance of authenticity. With a considerable degree of satisfaction, I concluded that things were looking even worse for Ellman and Casterbridge Hospital. It would only take a critical report from an independent expert for them to cave in and admit liability. There would then be a quick out-of-court settlement once damages were agreed. Whether disciplinary action would then be taken against Ellman would be a matter outside my control. In my opinion he should be struck off and banged up, but I would think that, wouldn't I? The other big question was whether I would ever find out what had really been going on. I very much hoped so, because it was truth and justice that I was really after, although I certainly wouldn't say no to the money – about £15,000 was being mentioned.

While I was combing through my notes, Bentham and Carr were briefing my independent expert, a top London gynaecologist. Unfortunately he decided he did not have time to deal with my complex case, so another apparently equally eminent expert was appointed, a Mr Andrew Jessop. When Bentham's secretary phoned me with this news, I had a vague feeling I'd heard the name before, but couldn't think in what context. So where had I seen the name Jessop recently, other than on camera shops? Of course! At the City and Royal Hospital. He was one of the other gynaecologists in the large and prestigious gynaecological oncology department. He and Prof Shaw would be close colleagues. As I strongly suspected that Shaw had made it his business to get the low-down on my case, I wondered how truly independent Jessop would turn out to be? I phoned Bentham's secretary asking her to tell him about this close connection. Would it matter? Presumably Bentham did not consider it an issue, as Jessop was duly instructed to go through my notes and prepare a report.

CHAPTER 17

Although I had had my MRI scan on the 14th of January, I didn't see Prof Shaw to discuss the findings until 26th of February. I think this might have been because he had tried to get me back to Casterbridge Hospital until he realised that I was having none of it, and wanted my case based entirely at the City and Royal. He was stuck with me, whether he liked it or not, and I had the feeling he didn't like it. I felt sure he knew, possibly more by deduction than by direct information, that my treatment at Casterbridge Hospital had been very unsatisfactory in some way. Quite understandably, he didn't want to get involved. Yet I was now regarding him as my only hope for ever getting my problems sorted out. Somehow I wanted him to have an accurate picture of my medical history, but at the same time I didn't want to antagonise him.

As face-to-face consultations always seemed so restricted in time – if you managed half an hour you had done extremely well – I thought the best thing was to write him a letter and include an accurate chronology of my medical history. So on the 10th of February I spent most of the day at my word processor. I explained that because of the three-year deadline, I had had to commence legal action for clinical negligence against Casterbridge Hospital concerning the 2000 operations. I assured him that the action would not extend to the City and Royal. I added that in the circumstances, I did not want further treatment at Casterbridge Hospital. Then I went on to describe my current symptoms, mainly frequent diarrhoea, and to question the incurable cancer diagnosis. I explained I had been doing some research in a medical dictionary and had come across hydatid disease, which causes cysts in various parts of the body. I explained that Mike had suffered a cyst on his pancreas which had necessitated two operations in 2000 and 2001. Could we have both contracted this disease during our travels? It can be caught from working dogs in sheep rearing areas, and can lie dormant for some years. We had been to New Zealand twice, and to iffy areas like South America, Africa and China. I had spent time on a sheep farm in Australia in 1973. Perhaps all this was a long shot, but I wanted Shaw to keep an open mind, and I felt it was desirable that he was aware of the extent of my foreign travel so that unusual diseases were not dismissed. I also mentioned that I thought further surgery was probably going to be necessary, but that at this stage I could not agree to the removal of my rectum.

I prepared a brief gynaecological history with exact dates starting on the 31st of May 1981. I did not go into any speculation or accusations about 'foreign objects' - I just stated what had been done (or not done) and what I had been told. The facts would speak for themselves, and Shaw could draw his own conclusions.

I received a prompt and informative reply, which impressed me. After all, Prof Shaw must be a very busy man, probably with a thriving private practice as well as NHS and academic work. If only I had received such courtesy from other consultants. Now I was even more determined to stay under him, which I supposed would mean agreeing to whatever he suggested. The letter made it clear that I must not dismiss chemotherapy, and that surgery would only be undertaken if I did agree to the removal of my rectum, if necessary.

Mike accompanied me to the consultation at the City and Royal on the 26th of February. The room was bursting at the seams - Mike and me, Prof Shaw, Dr Galton, Sally, and a foreign doctor who was observing. At least there were plenty of witnesses for what was to be discussed.

Prof Shaw's manner seemed a little different. He had never been other than polite and professional, but had sometimes come across as a little brusque. Now, somehow, he seemed warmer and more sympathetic, and more sure about the facts of my case. I think my letter had done some good.

"So how are you feeling, Mrs Bland?" he began when everyone was settled.

"It's a pretty shitty existence," I replied. "I'm on the loo every hour or two, day and night. I'm very loose, with a lot of mucus."

Shaw scribbled away in my file. "And what about the water works?"

"A bit slow. I must be like a man with a prostate problem."

Shaw looked at Dr Galton and grinned slightly. Did one of them have a prostate problem? They both looked in their late fifties. Mike had been afflicted around that age.

"The MRI scan shows the mass is pressing on your right ureter. We'll have to keep an eye on that because it could cause kidney damage," Shaw explained. He glanced at the scan report. "It's gone down since we drained off all that fluid, but there's still something there, very low down on the rectum. That's what's causing the bowel problems, and it's not going to get any better. Any pain?"

"Some bowel pain, but paracetamol and voltarol keeps it under control."

"So we must decide how we're going to treat this mass. Would you like to come in here?" He turned to Dr Galton.

"You could have chemotherapy. This would best be done at Casterbridge under Dr Oswald. But I would say there's only a thirty per cent chance it would be effective."

"I don't think it's worth trying then," I replied, "seeing it would make me feel worse than I am already. I'm still waiting to hear whether my cells are suitable for this octeotride treatment. Dr Oswald sent them off in late October. Surely I should have heard something by now."

Dr Galton and Prof Shaw exchanged what I interpreted as shifty glances.

"I shouldn't place any hope in that direction," Dr Galton said without further explanation. Questions flitted through my head. Why had I not received the result of the tests on my cells? Why had Oswald recommended investigating a treatment which his superior, the man who had trained him, appeared to be rejecting? Before I could say anything, Prof Shaw took over.

"I really think surgery offers the best chance for long-term remission."

"Yes, so do I," I agreed. "But I don't want to have a permanent colostomy. A temporary one, maybe, but not permanent. Couldn't you remove what you can, and then perhaps chemo could deal with the rest?"

"Until I open you up, I don't know what I'll be faced with. Scans only tell you so much. I simply wouldn't be prepared to operate with any kind of restrictions imposed on me. It wouldn't be in your best interest. You must trust me to do my best for you once I'm operating, although I must warn you that I might not be able to do anything. You would have to accept that as well."

The room fell silent. Everyone seemed to be looking at me.

"But a colostomy would be such a disability," I said.

"It wouldn't," Shaw replied rather sternly.

"You would lead a completely normal life," Sally assured me. "People with them work, travel, and do sports. I can arrange for a local stoma nurse to visit you and explain more about them."

Perhaps I was being unreasonably pessimistic. Terry Sutton had told me that he had heard the Queen Mother had had a colostomy. If true, it certainly hadn't stopped her leading an active and happy life.

"Well, I can't go on as I am," I concluded. "I suppose I must agree to surgery with no restrictions."

Prof Shaw looked relieved. "I think you've made the right decision," he said.

Sally escorted us out of the consulting room and we sat in the waiting area while she arranged a date for the operation. There appeared to be no great urgency. Unlike most ovarian cancers, mine appeared to be virtually dormant. It seemed the accumulation of fluid was the cause of most of my problems rather than the growth of the tumour. Neither was there any sign that the cancer was spreading. Indeed, there even seemed to be an element of doubt as to the very presence of active cancer cells. I felt that despite all the scans and tests, my insides were still a bit of a mystery to all concerned, and my treatment in the past further confused matters.

"I've arranged the op for the 8th of May," Sally said, approaching with a bundle of consent forms and the like. We'll need to do further tests and scans before then, and keep an eye on you, especially the kidney function."

"How long will I be in hospital?"

"About three weeks is the norm if you have a colostomy. It's quite a serious op. Perhaps a little less than that if you do well."

Sally was very down-to-earth and efficient. She really knew her job and seemed to have great empathy with her patients. Prof Shaw was lucky to have such good assistance. In fact, his whole team worked smoothly, and I put that down to good leadership from the top. Prof Shaw struck me as the sort of man who wouldn't stand for any nonsense from his colleagues or from the hospital management, neither, for that matter, from his patients. But he wasn't a bully like I suspected Ellman was. Shaw was in control because his competence and efficiency was respected and valued. I felt he had formed his own opinion about my case, but whatever he knew or suspected, I wasn't going to hear about it. He was a doctor; he had made it clear that he did not want to become embroiled in legal actions, so he would keep his mouth shut however disgusted he was by the actions of his colleagues. Anyway, I felt in safe hand under Prof Shaw.

"Do you think I've made the right decision?" I asked Mike as we travelled home on the coach. He had been very quiet during the consultation, knowing that he was there principally to witness proceedings.

"Yes. You should have agreed to surgery long ago. Let's hope it isn't too late now."

"Shaw would have fitted me in sooner if he thought things were going down hill fast. I reckon he knows something he's not telling me."

"Maybe, but I still think he'll do what's best for you."

"Well, I can't go on as I am. I suppose having a colostomy bag will be better than running to the loo every hour or so." I got up and made my way to the smelly little toilet at the back of the coach.

Now that the decision had been made, I felt more relaxed. A local stoma care nurse visited me and showed me bags and leaflets. She even arranged for me to talk on the phone to a lady who had had a colostomy many years ago and was leading a normal life including lots of foreign travel. My worries and fears started to recede.

Meanwhile legal matters proceeded slowly but steadily. Mr Andrew Jessop, the independent expert, needed to see me, so on the 5th of March Mike and I made another trip to London to see him at his private consulting rooms in Harley Street. I'd never been there before. Only very rich people frequent Harley Street. You could hardly move for the nearly new Jags, BMWs, and hulking great 4x4s. These doctors were doing all right because in addition to their outrageous private fees, most of them also got big fat salaries from the NHS for the set number of hours they slummed it in the real world.

The waiting room was all carpets, leather sofas, and the day's broadsheets, a far cry from the thinly padded benches and ancient copies of 'Woman's Weekly' in your average NHS waiting area. And we didn't have to wait long. No sooner had I picked up the 'Daily Telegraph' than we were being shown into an even more gracious consulting room. Mr Jessop, who appeared a good deal younger than Shaw, greeted us and proceeded to take a full medical history. He was very thorough, and so was I. When we got to the September 2000 operation, I mentioned all the strange events which had aroused my suspicions and had led me to the 'foreign object' theory. He noted everything down without comment. However, he seemed more interested in my on-going care after that operation, and although he made no observations, I think he was surprised that there were no further tests or treatment. After nearly two hours of questioning and note-taking, he asked to examine me. I lay on the screened-off couch in the corner of the room and he gently felt my tum. Fortunately he didn't want to do an internal examination.

At last he was satisfied that he had all the information he needed for the report. Probably quite correctly, he gave little away as to whether his findings would support my case. Proving my 'foreign object' theory was never going to be possible. It was more a question of looking at every aspect of my care, and perhaps drawing conclusions from the overall picture. As Mike and I took the tube back to the coach station, I wondered how much the report was going to cost. As the complexity of my case was revealed, the fees were rocketing, and there was no guarantee I would win my case and therefore have my legal costs paid as well as receiving damages. I was prepared to lose £10,000. I wasn't poor, but neither was I stinking rich. If more than £10,000 were to disappear, I would begin to notice it. If ever the outcome of the case was in serious doubt, I would have to stop throwing good money after bad. As things stood at the moment, it was worth continuing. I felt myself that there was more than enough evidence of some kind of wrong-doing what with the faked histology report and altered notes. That sort of thing just couldn't be ignored – it was all part of the cover-up.

"If we're going to get the seven o'clock coach, we're going to have to move," Mike said, abruptly bringing me out of my musings. We charged through Victoria Station and on to the coach terminal, boarding the Casterbridge coach with seconds to spare.

CHAPTER 18

Nothing happened through most of March. Legal matters could not move forwards until we had received Jessop's report. Healthwise, I seemed to be fairly stable. The constant diarrhoea continued and I experienced a certain amount of pain. I consumed paracetamol tablets like smarties, but fortunately the maximum safe dose was usually effective and did not cause any side effects. I could lead a normal life, and I became an expert on the location of public loos in the areas in which I travelled. Mentally, I told myself that I had accepted the situation, but had I? At times the thought of a colostomy bag still horrified me. My friends were sometimes subjected to earfuls of my doubts and fears as well as poor, long-suffering Mike. One Scrabble Club friend, Lena, who was in possession of such quick wits and devastating logic that she regularly cleaned up on TV game shows until she was banned, came out with the following: "So it's have a bag or die of cancer – it's a no-brainer, isn't it?"

That shut me up. She was right, of course, assuming the facts were right. But did I have cancer? Terry Sutton continued to express his doubts. When the solicitor finally obtained the latest notes from the City and Royal, I was able to read a letter Prof Shaw had written to Dr Galton after he had received my letter. In it he quite openly admitted his on-going confusion, and although he appeared not to think I had hydatid disease, he did mention 'some form of pseudomyomatous peritonei with falsely encapsulated fluid and mucin within the pelvis'.

Because there had been no spread of the disease, it seemed my case was unusual. All the strange terminology caused me to reach for my family health encyclopedia. I already knew that 'pseudo' meant 'false', so I looked for 'myomatous'. I found 'myoma', which is a non-cancerous tumour which can affect intestinal muscle. I already knew that the peritoneum is a skin that covers all the intestines and sort of holds everything together. So it seemed that Prof Shaw was wondering if I had a non-cancerous tumour that was causing fluid to form in the peritoneum. This would explain why he was suggesting the cancer was perhaps dormant, and why chemotherapy was not being strongly recommended. It really did seem that Casterbridge Hospital had made the cancer diagnosis without firm evidence. But I had to admit that I didn't really understand Prof Shaw's highly medical language. It was one specialist communicating with another. I was never meant to see such a letter. In general, reading one's medical notes is not a practice to be recommended.

The City and Royal notes revealed something else that was rather interesting and encouraging. During December, after the unexpected findings of the biopsy, Prof Shaw had asked Casterbridge Hospital to send slides of the material taken from my ovaries in 1981 and 2000. I remember him telling me that he wanted it re-examined in the City and Royal pathology lab. A junior doctor had noted in my file that Casterbridge had sent these vital, irreplaceable tissue samples by second class post – close to Christmas, and at a time when it was widely known that packages were going missing from London sorting offices. It was almost as if they wanted the samples to get lost. Surely they should have used an ambulance or hospital car going to London, or a medical courier service. The fact that a junior doctor had seen fit to write 'by second class post' suggested it was unusual. So what was going on? Bearing in mind that the fabricated 1981 histology report related to the 1981 samples, my suspicions were now in overdrive.

I found the City and Royal lab reports on the 1981, 2000, and 2002 material. Once more I was faced with impenetrable medical jargon, so once more the family health encyclopedia came down from the bookshelf, but it was of little use in interpreting 'focal minor invasion and surface involvement'. However, I was able to conclude that my first cancer in 1981 had been very early, the term 'micro-invasion' suggesting it could only be seen under a microscope. In 2000 the cells taken from the right ovary remnant were exactly the same as those seen in 1981. Presumably this was because the radiotherapy had stopped further development of cancer cells, but the changes that had already taken place remained, but in a dormant form. It appeared no cancerous cells had been found in the cyst on the left ovary which had been removed in 2000, nor in the part of the uterus which had been removed. The 2002 biopsy showed cells identical to those found in 1981 and 2000 in the right ovary. So where exactly had the biopsy been taken from? The word 'borderline' was frequently used, although it appeared that over a period of 21 years, what cancer there might have been in me had never progressed beyond this rather iffy status. I began to realise that it might well be impossible for doctors to say definitely whether or not a patient has cancer. Perhaps millions of people are in an iffy state for years without ever knowing it because they don't have any symptoms. Prof Shaw had even suggested that something else might carry me off before the cancer did.

But all this study and thought did raise three questions in my mind.

Firstly, why did Casterbridge Hospital, or, rather, Dr Oswald, make a diagnosis of incurable and virtually untreatable cancer based on a 21-year-old sample showing borderline cancer, a two and a half-year-old sample showing no change in the intervening period, and nothing more recent? That was unbelievable.

Secondly, why had the cells showing borderline changes

remained identical from 1981 to 2000? During that time they would have been subjected to ten weeks of radiation, and to nearly 19 years of continuing life during which further changes might reasonably have been expected. Yet the word used by the pathologist was 'identical'. I remembered that in January 2000 I had been told by Ellman's registrar that the 1981 tissue samples had probably been destroyed – quite likely given the time period. Certainly they had not been re-examined by Ellman. Perhaps they should have been. Then an appalling thought occurred. Perhaps the 1981 samples weren't really from 1981. Perhaps they *had* been destroyed, possibly in error, and material taken in 2000 from the 'right ovary remnant' had been deliberately mislabelled as from 1981. Then, obviously, the two specimens would be the same. As soon as this thought formed, I found myself dismissing it. Probably presentation and staining techniques for tissue samples would have changed between 1981 and 2000, and any pathologist would have noticed if the 1981 samples weren't the real thing. Or would he? It seemed no one had noticed a fabricated histology report, except me. If you're not on the look-out for something, you don't necessarily notice it. Then there was this 'closing ranks' thing. I began to wonder if I was becoming paranoid. However, given what I had already found out, and given that I was aware that I might be going too far in this instance, I was reasonably confident that I was still rational – suspicious, but not paranoid.

The third question was why I had developed cystic material when it appeared the cancer cells were dormant. Was a completely separate disease the cause of the problem? Was the cancer a complete red herring? I had felt all along that the doctors had been jumping to conclusions, and that really I should be having a wider range of tests. I believed Prof Shaw to be more open-minded, but I knew he was now likely to keep up the cancer pretence so that I wouldn't be able to take action against Dr Oswald.

By the middle of March my health was deteriorating again. My weight increased and my legs became swollen, suggesting fluid retention. It seemed possible my kidneys weren't working properly because of pressure on the ureters, the tubes between the kidneys and bladder. Scans had shown there was some pressure on the right side one. I started to get a slight watery vaginal discharge, similar to what I had had after the biopsy had been taken. Perhaps now more fluid had built up and was spontaneously discharging. Better out than in, I thought. Matters reached a head in the early hours of Sunday the 23rd of March. I woke up soaked in watery blood. Mike immediately called an ambulance and at 4.30am I found myself being wheeled into the A and E department at Casterbridge Hospital. It was like entering the lions' den. I just didn't want to be treated in a hospital I was suing. But there was no choice. After all, Casterbridge A and E was less than a mile from my home.

I was left on a trolley in a cubicle. A nurse monitored me, particularly my blood pressure, but didn't seem to be especially concerned about me when I explained what I thought was going on. Although I had been admitted at 4.30am, I did not see a doctor until 11.30am. I thought that was appalling. It was explained to me that a child badly injured in a road accident had been admitted at about the same time and was in far greater need of urgent attention. But I was still appalled – there seemed to be serious understaffing. Mike stayed with me most of the time, but there was little he could do. I was soaking one incontinence pad after another, but the loss was more fluid than blood. I also needed to urinate frequently. In various ways all the stored-up fluid seemed to be pouring out of my body.

By the time I saw a rather harassed young doctor, the discharge was subsiding. He seemed to agree with my own diagnosis of a spontaneous release of fluid which had been building up over the last few months. I was discharged at

1pm and told to see my GP the following day. Mike came and picked me up. Once home, I went straight to the bathroom scales. I had been monitoring my weight almost daily, so I knew exactly what I had weighed the previous day. My weight had dropped from 13 stone 2 pounds to 12 stone 2 pounds in a matter of hours. It just showed how much fluid weighs, and also that my slow weight gain had had nothing to do with overeating.

I saw Dr Wilson on the Tuesday, and explained what had happened, mentioning the drastic weight loss. He was concerned and sent a fax to Prof Shaw. The next day Dr Baxter, Prof Shaw's fellow (the teaching hospital term for a registrar) phoned me to check how I was feeling. I had met Dr Baxter while at the City and Royal and had found him very pleasant. I had a vague feeling he was being more open and honest with me than Shaw was, probably because he had no knowledge of the impending legal action, as far as I was aware.

"I'm feeling a lot better," I told him.

"I would expect that if more pus has been released," he said.

Pus? According to Shaw it was some kind of mucus accumulating in my pelvis, not pus. Yet Dr Baxter had performed the biopsy. He was the one who had collected the yuk which had unexpectedly poured out of me. He had called it pus. Notes from the City and Royal mentioned 'frank pus'. The word 'frank' used in a medical context means 'unmistakeable'. Hadn't they then spent the next few days pumping me full of strong intravenous antibiotics? Whatever else was going on, I obviously had pelvic infection, quite possibly caused by botched surgery under Ellman. For some reason Shaw seemed to be brushing this under the carpet, whereas Baxter was far more up-front about it. Was there a real difference of opinion between the two of them? That was all I needed. I suspected it was more a question of spin.

Possibly I was suffering from both infection and fluid accumulation. Was one causing the other, or were they unrelated conditions?

After a few more questions Dr Baxter decided no further action was necessary. I was instructed to take things easy and call the doctor at the slightest sign of further trouble. I carried on as normal. Terry Sutton was giving me regular tests and some electro-magnetic treatment which he thought might be effective against my hardly-there cancer. The problem was, it would take time, about two months Terry estimated.

"But I'm having the op on the 8th of May," I said. "Not much more than a month now."

"Well, you have a choice," he replied. "You can go ahead with the op and risk a permanent colostomy, or ask for the op to be postponed while we give this treatment a chance. By June we'll have a better idea of how it's working. I know what I'd do, but whatever you decide, I'll do what I can for you."

"A colostomy is so final," I replied. "Obviously I don't want it if it can be avoided."

"I would agree. You may not be able to avoid it, but it's worth a try."

"Prof Shaw isn't going to like it if I cancel. It all probably takes a lot of planning. I don't want to get on the wrong side of him."

"I could write to him explaining what I'm doing, and suggest a postponement so long as he considers it to be safe. How about that?"

"Yes, it might be a good idea. Let me see what sort of letter you'd write, then I'll think about it. You see, I know Shaw has no time for complementary medicine. He knows about the treatment I've been having under you. He's not exactly hostile, but he just thinks it doesn't do any good. I think he takes the view that if I think it's doing me good, it possibly is."

"The placebo effect," Terry explained. "Perhaps he doesn't realise that certain homeopathic and other treatments work effectively on animals, and they, as far as we know, aren't susceptible to the placebo effect."

"I know that. But you'll never get conventional doctors to be more open-minded, especially not the older ones like Shaw."

Terry and I had had many long discussions about the role of complementary medicine. He worked on the international cutting edge in the field, often travelling to seminars in both Russia and the USA. I was lucky to know him. However, I myself remained sceptical about some aspects of his work, and I always viewed his treatment as complementary rather than alternative. Now he was suggesting that I did consider it as an alternative to surgery.

Before I could make a decision on the matter, I had to go to the City and Royal for another MRI scan. Shaw was obviously intent on finding out as much as possible before cutting me open, and quite right too. Just before I departed, a copy of the independent expert's report landed on the front doormat with a covering letter from Bentham. It was not encouraging. He had not had time to read the twenty-page report, but had read the conclusion. He wrote, 'I have read the conclusion and I note that in summary he does not feel there is a strong basis for a claim of medical negligence against Casterbridge Hospital NHS Trust'. He asked me to read through the report very carefully, let him have my comments, and consider my position. This was a blow. The other nasty shock was the independent expert's bill - £2,700. That was the cost of an exotic long-haul holiday. (I tended to value everything in terms of what sort of holiday it would buy.) I was now very close to the £10,000 cut-off point as regards legal fees.

Once the coach was steadily cruising up the motorway I took out the report and a pen to mark anything I thought worthy of comment. I just hoped the language wasn't going to be too technical as I obviously hadn't humped along my dictionary and medical encyclopedia.

It was evident from very early on in the report that Jessop was placing great importance on the cancer aspect of my case. I suppose that was understandable given that he was principally a gynaecological oncologist. He recognised the complex nature of my case, given the previous history of cancer nearly nineteen years before the 2000 operation. His first criticism of my case was that pre-operative investigation seemed a little inadequate in the circumstances, and that post-operative follow-up should have been more thorough with more scans and CA125 blood tests, and a multidisciplinary team discussion. My immediate assumption was that these things had not taken place because Ellman was hiding something. After all, Casterbridge Hospital had a specialist cancer centre. They were well able at that stage to give me thorough on-going care, so why hadn't they? The report was revealing new aspects of negligence, and in my eyes was strengthening my case. So why the unexpected conclusion? I scribbled 'this is damning' by the 'comment' paragraph, and read on.

Jessop had similar adverse comments about the pre-parations for the September 2000 operation. There should have been a CT or MRI scan, and the tests on the waterworks which had been requested but never carried out, were also important. There should also have been a multidisciplinary team discussion. It seemed that Jessop thought the likely surgery at that stage would be difficult and complex and that the surgical team were ill-prepared for it. That was hardly surprising, I thought cynically, when all they were going to do was remove a swab or something. You hardly needed the elaborate preparations detailed in the report. Surely the lack of preparation in a hospital with adequate resources to handle my case was a reason for suspicion. It seemed that Jessop did not see it that way, although I was pleased to see that my own theory about a swab being left in me had been mentioned. However, it was pointed out there was no objective evidence for this. Among other rather critical comments, he expressed surprise that no biopsy was obtained. He pointed out that this was essential for my future management. If only, I thought, he would take on board the 'foreign object' scenario, he would understand why.

Jessop went on to mention his surprise that at the following multidisciplinary meeting it was decided to simply keep me under observation. He was concerned and surprised that there were no notes about the discussion leading to this decision. I wasn't surprised at all, seeing I suspected that the meeting had never taken place. Jessop had not considered that a possible scenario. Towards the end of the report he briefly mentioned the fabricated 1981 histology report, commenting that he would have expected it to have been generated directly from the microfiche on which it was almost certainly stored, and not retyped from what appeared to be a handwritten record. He appeared to be very non-committal on the issue, recognising that things did not appear quite right, but not making any comment on what might be wrong. I felt he knew, or suspected, much more than he was letting on.

His final conclusion was that my care in 2000 and the lack of suitable on-going care was not ideal in some respects but that it did not amount to negligence. Had the care been better, it might not have made any difference to how my disease had developed, the implication being that mine was a pretty hopeless case from the beginning. I simply didn't believe that, and nothing that was said to me in 2000 suggested that might be the case.

The coach had now reached the London suburbs and was making jerky progress through the traffic. I couldn't read any more so I stared out of the window at the river as we crawled along Chelsea Embankment. I tried to review things. It seemed that the Jessop report had introduced yet another possible scenario, so I now had four to choose from:-

One – my own, the 'foreign object' theory.

Two – Ellman's, the 'reactive swelling' explanation.

Three – Oswald's, Ellman missed the mass during the first op.

Four – Jessop's, The mass grew between the operations.

Of these four possibilities, Jessop's (although he was by far the best-qualified to understand the situation) was the most unlikely. He had overlooked the fact that my bowel symptoms had not progressively worsened between the 2000 operations. They had developed quite suddenly and, if anything, had improved slightly over the months. It also seemed most unlikely that a rapidly growing mass should not continue to grow, but scans had shown it had expanded only very slightly between August 2000 and September 2002. I still thought my own theory was the most likely. In fact, now that the report had pointed out what should have been done following both operations, my suspicions of cover-up had strengthened. There had to be a reason why I didn't have the correct follow-up, and the plan of deception was the reason.

At the City and Royal I spent another boring hour or so in the noisy MRI scanner. I tried to doze, but my brain was in overdrive. I knew that my 'foreign object' theory could never be proved. At best, the evidence was circumstantial. It was probably not going to stand up in a court case. However, the Jessop report had opened up another possible avenue – lack of care amounting to negligence in the post-operative management of my case. If it could be proved that, on balance, I would have been cured of cancer or could expect long-term remission following the appropriate treatment, I had a case. It was just a question of getting Jessop's mealy-mouthed conclusions beefed up a bit. It might also depend on what exactly was going on in my body at the moment, which all seemed a bit of a mystery. Everything seemed such a mess. It seemed that if I was to win my case I was going to have to run with a falsehood, i.e. inadequate management of developing cancer. I would have to put all ideas of foreign objects right out of my mind. Ironically, this twist of events made my case much more serious. If, indeed, I now had incurable cancer, if, indeed, I would lose my rectum, the damages would rocket if negligence was proved. Something left in me after an operation was trivial by comparison. But I knew Ellman would never own up to this as it would mean he would have to admit to a deliberate cover-up. It would be better for him to run with the negligent after-care scenario. What a tangled web!

After another CA125 blood test, I returned to Casterbridge, anxious to prepare my comments for Bentham on the Jessop report. I wanted to convince him that although my 'foreign object' theory could not be proved, and could not be used as the basis for a successful action, the report pointed out sufficient incidences of neglect to provide evidence for an action of negligence. The lack of suitable scans and follow-up treatment appeared more than adequate proof.

My letter to Bentham came to six carefully argued pages with numerous references to the Jessop report. I pointed out minor, and mainly inconsequential errors before going on to the nitty-gritty. My first major point was that I was not referred to the cancer specialists at Casterbridge Hospital after the February 2000 operation because I believed Ellman was trying to hide something. I argued that he would be thoroughly familiar with the process for onward referral in the case of unexpected cancer found during an operation. I questioned why neither the GMC nor the expert used by the NHS complaints procedure had pointed out his poor, or even negligent, management of my case. I concluded that the complaints procedure was crap – and that is the exact word I used.

Further points I raised included the lack of further scans or physical examinations until well over six months after the first operation, and how Ellman's letter after the first operation telling me further disease was very unlikely lulled me into a false sense of security. I then went on to question whether a multidisciplinary meeting had indeed taken place after the second operation, saying this would explain why Jessop could find no notes about it. I also pointed out that preparation for my second operation seemed unduly rushed, and did not include a multidisciplinary discussion despite the fact that the operation was possibly going to be difficult. Another point was that previous investigation under the complaints procedure had stated that an ultrasound scan was adequate at that stage, whereas Jessop had stated that CT or MRI scans were necessary. I felt that lots of little points were building up into a great big highly unsatisfactory and suspicious scenario. I hoped very much that Bentham and Carr would take the same view.

I received a very prompt reply from Bentham which contained both good and bad news. The good news was that he emphasised that the Jessop report was in draft form, and that my barrister could suggest to Jessop that certain aspects of it could be strengthened to help prove my case for negligence. The bad news was that as things stood at the moment, I did not have a sound case. Whether Ellman's non-action amounted to negligence appeared to be questionable, and even if it had been, there was the problem of whether there was a causative link between this negligence and my current condition. In other words, it was likely I would have developed inoperable cancer whatever Ellman had or hadn't done. Personally, I felt that the law would be on my side on that issue. Every lay person had it firmly in their head that the earlier cancer is diagnosed and treated, the better the outcome. Doctors would have to agree that, in general, that was indeed correct. Therefore the balance of probability was that any developing cancer would have been caught much sooner if I had had the right sort of scans at the right time. I felt quite pleased with my reasoning. Perhaps I should have done law at university, rather than geography.

Bentham's letter was full of dire warnings about the legal bills I would run up if I proceeded further. The next major step would be a case conference with Jessop, Carr, Bentham, and myself in Carr's chambers in London. It would probably last for at least two hours in addition to all the preparatory work and travel time. I did a few quick sums; it could cost over £5,000, meaning that my total spend would greatly top the £10,000 limit I had had in mind. Was it worth going on? Bentham didn't appear to think so. He asked for my instructions in writing if I did decide to continue.

I felt like a gambler must feel after a heavy loss. The instinct is to continue in the hope of regaining the loss and going on to win. That is the road to ruin and bankruptcy. It is often better to cut and run, retreat and lick your wounds. But this action wasn't a gamble. I wanted truth, not money. Would I ever get to the truth? Was it worth shelling out yet more to try? Would I really miss another five thousand or so lopped off my savings? The answer was 'no'. I craved truth, knowledge, and peace of mind above anything else. The action would continue.

I instructed Bentham to seek an extension of time from the court for the case preparation. He would then send the Jessop report to Jeremy Carr for his opinion on how matters should proceed.

It seemed fairly clear that the case was now about my inadequate treatment in connection with the cancer threat. I could forget about 'foreign objects'. In fact, if it could be shown that I had developed incurable cancer through negligence, the possible damages would be far in excess of anything I might have received from the 'foreign object' scenario. I might as well keep quiet about that, especially as I could never prove it. The case had taken an unexpected turn, but it seemed this was to my advantage. The Jessop report directed matters very much along the 'developing cancer' road. Although I believed this was a contrived cover-up based on very flimsy evidence, it seemed it would be to my advantage to run with this lie. If Ellman found himself hoisted by his own petard it would serve him bloody-well right.

I discussed all this with my friend Amy, the retired medical secretary, when I gave her a lift to the Scrabble club.

"I still think the 'something left in me' scenario is the correct one," I said. "It explains why I didn't get the monitoring I should have done in 2000. But at the same time I've got to take on board the fact that if something had gone wrong in the op, it would have been better, and presumably safer, for Ellman to have owned up to it and put it right instead of embarking on elaborate subterfuge. I can't understand that."

Amy sat beside me, looking very thoughtful.

"I remember reading something about Ellman in the local paper," she said, frowning as she tried to recall the details. "It was about a case brought by some woman – he hadn't done something he should have done – I think she won."

I was all ears. "When was this?"

"A year or two ago – quite a long time ago, anyway."

"And it was in the Casterbridge Clarion?"

"Yes. I didn't see it, but a friend gave me the cutting as she knew I'd be interested."

"Have you still got it?"

"No, I threw it away."

I resolved immediately to track down the story. I knew someone who worked on the editorial side of the Clarion. He'd have easy access to back numbers and, no doubt, to some fancy computer-based index system for the retrieval of old news. No way was I going to spend hours scanning old editions in the library. So a few days later I had a word with my friend. It would only be a few minutes' work for him. The very next day an envelope containing a photocopied front page of the Clarion was popped through my letterbox. It was dated the 16th of March 2000 and the headline was 'Woman wins damages'. I read the report avidly:

'In a case of medical negligence at Casterbridge County Court Mrs Emma Bentham...' I stopped reading and almost fell off my perch. Bentham! There were hardly any Benthams in Casterbridge. I had noticed that when I had once looked in the phone directory to see if I could find where Joseph Bentham lived (he was ex-directory). So who was this Emma Bentham – his wife, his mother, aunt, cousin? There was a strong chance that there was a relationship. I read on: '....Mrs Emma Bentham has won substantial damages. The defendants, Casterbridge Hospital NHS Trust, settled out of court after a hearing lasting half a day during which overwhelming evidence of negligence was presented by the prosecution.'

The report was quite detailed, explaining that James Ellman, the consultant gynaecologist treating Mrs Bentham, had, it appeared, virtually forced his registrar, Dr Hick, to perform an operation on the lady that she knew she was incapable of carrying out. Not surprisingly, the operation was botched, leaving Mrs Bentham with some kind of permanent bladder disorder. It seemed that Ellman had not even been present in the theatre to supervise. It was indeed appalling negligence. How had Dr Hick felt? No wonder she had gone out of her way to alert me to what she believed had happened in my case. Ellman was a bully, and she wanted him to get found out. Then there was the timing. The case would have been hanging over Ellman when he operated on me in February 2000. Was his mind on the job? No doubt the Shipman verdict, announced the previous day, had made him dwell on his own case. Then he made another error at a time when his performance must have been under scrutiny. He was like a driver with nine points on his licence being flashed by a speed camera. Elaborate cover-up was the only way he was going to save his career.

I felt I had just fitted the last piece into a particularly difficult jigsaw puzzle. It was great! At last I had a motive for my scenario. It was the possibility I had vaguely considered, but now here was evidence in black and white! I thought back to Bentham's remarks about Ellman's incompetence when we had first met. I remembered the almost unprofessional vehemence he'd shown. I felt sure this Mrs Bentham was a relation. I certainly had the right solicitor.

I showed Mike the newspaper report.

"That explains quite a lot," he said, "but it's not going to make any difference to the way your case is progressing. Jeremy Carr needs to show your follow-up treatment was negligent, that's all. Why it was is neither here nor there. You'll never get the truth. You've got to get that into your head."

Despite Mike's views, I felt happier. The one flaw in my 'foreign object' scenario had been removed. I was surer than ever that the scenario was substantially correct.

CHAPTER 19

I knew there would now be a hiatus in the legal proceedings. Jeremy Carr would spend some time preparing his advice in the light of the Jessop report. I was going to be out of action for a few weeks after my impending operation. It was time to concentrate on health issues rather than legal matters

Since the spontaneous outpouring of fluid at the end of March, I had felt quite well. Terry Sutton continued to treat me, and according to him, I was indeed improving. He really thought he could shrink the tumour if he had more time.

"Would you consider asking for the op to be postponed?" he asked me once more.

"I couldn't. It's all booked. Prof Shaw wouldn't be at all pleased."

"He'd soon fill the slot with someone else if he has sufficient notice. Remember, if you lose your rectum, that's it. If I have another month or so, that might not happen. Even if you do ultimately need an operation, it might not be so serious. Isn't it worth a try?"

I had to agree that it was.

"Could you write to Prof Shaw explaining what you're doing? It would be better coming from you. But I don't think he's got much time for alternative treatments."

"I'll do that if it's what you'd like."

I knew I was taking a slight risk. I could deteriorate again and there was no knowing how long I might have to wait for another operation date. However, I had been encouraged by the result of a recent CA125 blood test at the City and Royal. It was down to 38 from a high of 439 in the previous November. Sally explained that it was now only fractionally above normal. It appeared that the high reading had been caused almost entirely by infection rather than cancer. Although it was always emphasised that the CA125 test was not always a good indicator of the presence or absence of cancer, Sally's manner encouraged me. The conventional medical view now appeared in line with Terry's –that if cancer was present, it was extremely borderline. No doubt this recent finding would persuade Prof Shaw that a postponement was safe.

It was now only a week before the operation, and before Terry could write the letter to Shaw, I had to go up to the City and Royal for pre-op checks. I saw Dr Baxter, Shaw's fellow.

"I'm feeling much better," I told him. "I'd like the operation postponed if it's safe to do so. I'm having alternative treatment, you see, and it's having some effect, but my therapist needs more time. He's going to write to Prof Shaw explaining things."

"I see. So you don't want to come in next week."

"No. I'm sorry it's such short notice. It's just that I don't want to lose my rectum if there's a chance of saving it."

Dr Baxter sat at his desk just looking at me. I'd taken him completely by surprise. "I'll have to discuss this with Prof right away." He fished a mobile out of his trouser pocket and left the room. I immediately felt guilty. Prof Shaw would hit the roof, as an operation like mine took quite a bit of planning. I could imagine the language that would pass between them about me. What had I done?

After a few minutes Dr Baxter returned, looking none too pleased.

"I've cancelled next week's op, but Prof is very concerned about pressure on you ureters – the tubes between your kidneys and bladder. If these stop working, you'd quickly become very ill as the body can't excrete toxins. We'll need to look at how they're functioning and make periodic checks on blood levels."

"Yes, I understand. If there's any danger of kidney problems, I suppose I'll have to have the operation."

Dr Baxter looked a little happier. Perhaps he realised I wasn't being totally stupid. He made arrangements for me to have a renogram, a test which would show how my water works were coping. I left the hospital feeling quite relieved that I hadn't been put under too much pressure to go ahead with the operation. It suggested that even Prof Shaw was moving away from the cancer diagnosis. I was finally as sure as I could be that he too was highly suspicious about what had been going on at Casterbridge Hospital, and that he now believed my version of events – not that he'd ever admit it.

Ten days later I travelled up to the City and Royal again for the renogram. Prof Shaw was very insistent that every test should be carried out by the City and Royal, and knowing what had been going on at Casterbridge, I couldn't blame him. However, it resulted in a lot of tedious travel up and down from London. As I was feeling fairly well, I decided to make better use of these trips. So after the tests, I walked all the way to the West End and managed to get a ticket for the matinee performance of 'Mama Mia'. I enjoyed it hugely, being a sad old Abba fan, and as I sang along with the rest of the audience, I couldn't help concluding that there wasn't much wrong with me except the need for rather frequent trips to the loo. Perhaps I'd be able to fit in some more shows after my hospital visits. Most would have the odd seat available on the day.

While at the City and Royal, I dropped a note for Prof Shaw into the gynae department, all full of apologies for messing him about by postponing the operation. I had to accept that Terry's treatment might not be fully effective, and that I would ultimately need the operation. I had to keep on the right side of him. Once I knew that Terry had also written to him, I wrote again, and for the first time I aired some of my suspicions about what had been going on at Casterbridge. The point I emphasised was that the mass somehow disappeared after the September 2000 operation, and that the mass now troubling me had only started to form in the summer of 2002. I suggested it could be a cyst or abscess caused by diverticular disease, pointing out that there were slight signs of this on the sigmoidoscopy performed in September 2000. I wondered whether the cancer diagnosis from Casterbridge had clouded the issue. I pointed out that what had gone on in September 2000 formed the major part of my legal action. I also admitted to getting cold feet about further surgery because I felt my case was still not fully understood, and because on my previous four trips to the operating theatre unexpected things had happened, and I couldn't face that happening again.

My expectation that legal matters would quieten down for a few weeks was soon proved wrong. Bentham wrote and asked me for a full and detailed statement of everything that had happened to me health-wise since the period covered by my previous statement, which had ended just before I first went to the City and Royal. Of course, an awful lot had happened, much of it very unexpectedly. I have always kept a diary, religiously recording everything I did during the day when I go to bed. It proved very useful for providing accurate dates and times for every event. Sometimes I would record in great detail what had happened or what doctors had said to me if I thought it might prove important. Bentham asked that my statement was backed up by photocopied pages from my diary for significant events. I think he was quite pleased that I was a bit obsessive when it came to recording my life. Mike had always teased me for noting down the same boring litany – shopped, did hovering, got lunch, played Scrabble, went to chess club, watched TV, etc. etc.

"I knew one day it would come in useful," I said.

Bentham also wanted me to start preparing a statement of losses and expenses. Assuming my case was successful, I would be able to claim these in addition to any damages I was awarded. Expenses were not too difficult. It was just a question of keeping an accurate record of travel costs, every single coach, tube, and taxi fare. It was surprising how they mounted up, what with the frequent trips to London. But when it came to losses, I was at a loss. For most people it would be loss of earnings, but I hadn't worked since April 2000. This was because Mike's ill-health had forced him into retirement, and when he had sold the practice to his partner, I lost my job in the practice. I neither needed nor wished for another job, as we lived comfortably on Mike's pensions and interest from our savings. I explained to Bentham that although I had stopped working soon after my first operation in 2000, it was not as a result of the operation.

"I appreciate your honesty," he said when we discussed things on the phone. "But you must think about other losses, perhaps the loss of your services to the household as you're principally a housewife. I expect you need household and garden help. No doubt you can't do as much as you used to. Are there any casual or part-time earnings you no longer have?"

"I sometimes give slide shows to clubs and groups. I've had to cancel some of them."

"Well, that's a loss. Try to give some figures to show what income you've lost. Remember too that if you have needed help around the home, that's an expense."

Bentham was obviously very used to calculating losses and expenses, and doing his best to exaggerate them, knowing that the other side would be doing their best to reduce them. It was all a good money-making game.

Through most of May I felt quite well, but it seemed the doctors were, in fact, very worried about me. At a much later date, as my case progressed, I eventually saw the correspondence which had passed between Prof Shaw and Dr Wilson, my GP. Shaw was extremely concerned about pressure on my ureters. He feared that even if he did get round to operating on me, it would be too late to do anything. Wilson was concerned about the increasing toxins in my blood, indicating that my kidneys weren't working properly. By the beginning of June I was quite ill, constantly being sick, and hardly able to stay awake. It was the build-up of creatinine and urea in my body – I was slowly poisoning myself. Something had to be done urgently. I was admitted to the urology department of Sandcliffe Hospital (all urology being dealt with at Casterbridge's neighbouring town) and placed under the care of Mr Rodd, the consultant urologist. He quickly deduced that my internal plumbing wasn't working, so external by-passes had to be rigged up. Under local anaesthetic small tubes (called nef tubes) were stuck directly into my kidneys, and attached to bags which collected the urine. So that I could wander about, I had a sort of elastic belt slung round my neck to which I could pin the bags, which soon filled up with liquid the colour of cherryade – the procedure having caused bleeding in the kidneys. It wasn't very comfortable having tubes sprouting out of my back, but at least I quite quickly felt a lot better, until I went down with a urinary infection, a common complication.

I told Mr Rodd that it was now obvious I would have to have the operation, as I didn't want to risk permanent kidney damage. He said he would get on to Prof Shaw, and that he would then consider putting stents into my ureters which would hold them open until I was over the operation.

Eventually I got this done, but I still wasn't peeing very well. A scan showed that my bladder wasn't draining out properly, no doubt due to pressure from the tumour, cyst, or whatever it was. I had to have a catheter put in, and that did the trick. So, at last, after seventeen days in Sandcliffe Hospital I was sent home with this catheter in which made sitting down very uncomfortable. Now it was a question of keeping in touch with the City and Royal and hoping that a new date would soon be available for the operation. This time I would go ahead with it – there was no alternative.

Back at home there was more correspondence from Bentham. There had been a delay in getting copies of my notes from the City and Royal. Bentham needed these to send to a company which would sort all my notes from all sources into a carefully organised and paginated file which would then become a sort of bible of reference for my barrister and for the defence. In a case as complicated as mine, which was now the concern of three hospitals, the professional expertise of a medical screening company was obviously a necessary expense.

The work was completed by the end of June and I received a bulky lever-arch file with all my medical notes filed and paginated in various sections. There was a brief summary of my medical history and an index to the various sections. After a little browsing, I was soon able to locate any specific document. In future any reference to a medical document would have to include the page number, so that all parties would know exactly what was being referred to. The company had been very thorough, and had attempted to identify possible missing documents. Like Professor Shaw, they seemed to have an uneasy feeling that here and there things didn't quite fit together. No doubt they were inclined to think that certain items had been 'lost', whereas I knew that certain tests and discussions, which everyone assumed had been carried out, never took place. Personally, I could not detect any missing notes. Copies of these notes were also sent to Jeremy Carr and Jessop so that they could prepare for the case conference. In view of my impending operation, and the likely possibility that its outcome could affect my case, it now seemed this conference would not be scheduled until the autumn. Bentham was already preparing to ask the court for a second four month time extension on account of my imminent operation.

Before the operation, Prof Shaw wanted to do another examination under anaesthetic. He obviously wanted to find out as much as he possibly could about my condition so that he could plan his surgery and not be faced with any unexpected situation. I admired his thoroughness. Because I had a catheter and was also suffering from bowel incontinence I was deemed too ill to travel up to London on public transport. I had a hospital car, which to my amazement was completely free. The first stage was another MRI scan, but as it would take a week or so to get the results, I was sent home again.

A week later I went up again and saw Prof Shaw. He explained that he wanted to get another biopsy and examine me under anaesthetic before definitely deciding what to do. The procedure was carried out the following day. Once again, the guided needle biopsy technique resulted in the release of a considerable amount of fluid from the cyst. They seemed unsure of whether they had any useful material. Anyway, from my point of view, the release of fluid was a good thing. I suggested I might now be able to pee normally, so they removed the catheter, and a few hours later I was urinating in the loo like a normal person again. What a relief!

Then I had yet another MRI scan to see what had happened now that more fluid had been drained off. A few days later I saw Prof Shaw again, and he seemed quite optimistic about everything.

"I'll operate next week on the 31st of July. Things are looking better than I feared. I would say there's only a twenty per cent chance you'll need a permanent colostomy, as I may be able to remove the mass from your rectum. However, it's a difficult situation, and it's impossible to know what's going to be necessary until I'm in there. You can only get a limited picture from a scan. You've got to understand that."

"Yes, I do, but I suppose it's quite good news. Do you think it's cancer? I hear my CA125 is up to 65."

"Sixty-five is only a little above normal, and not surprising given your recent kidney problems. The biopsy was inconclusive. I would say cancer is unlikely, but I can't rule it out. Everything I remove will be sent to pathology and tested, so you might have to wait for some while after the op before we can be sure one way or another. Anyway, even if I do find cancer, I think it will be in an early stage, and you'll be able to have some chemotherapy."

It was all reasonably encouraging news. As always, Prof Shaw was going through every possible eventuality and making sure I understood everything. I think he might have been erring on the side of optimism, but I expect it was in the back of his mind that I was going to get cold feet again. Perhaps, therefore, a little optimism was justified. At least the 'I might not be able to do anything' possibility no longer featured.

"I suggest you go home for a few days," he continued. "We'll have you back again on the 29th to get you ready for the op."

He briefly admired the tapestry of a ship in full sail I was working on, and with an encouraging smile he was gone. If only all doctors could be like Prof Shaw.

CHAPTER 20

The 29th of July started badly. I was due to present myself at the City and Royal after lunch. I understood that a car would call for me at 9am, as the journey to London could often take four hours or more. The car came at 6am. I was still fast asleep, and not packed. The driver had other people to collect en-route, so I had to send him on his way. What a total cock-up! Up until this, the car service had been reasonably OK, except that sometimes rather long and indirect routes were necessary to accommodate other passengers. I hoped this incident wasn't an omen. Later that morning I phoned the hospital to explain what had happened. Because I no longer had the catheter, I felt able to deal with public transport, so later on Mike dropped me at the coach station and I managed to get a seat to London. My only concession to my weakened state was a taxi rather than the tube on to the City and Royal.

I arrived around three o'clock, and the rest of the day was spent dealing with all the usual admission administration like being asked for the umpteenth time whether I used things like glasses, dentures, hearing aids, or walking aids.

"No one ever looks at these forms," the bored nurse admitted as she filled in the extensive questionnaire. "But it all has to be done and filed away."

I was only allowed a very light tea, and the following day I would be limited to drinks only. It was going to be necessary to get my digestive system completely cleared out. The next day I had an X-ray done of the water works, and then I met the specialist stoma nurse. In case I did need a stoma, which is the place where the end of the bowel is brought out to the surface of the abdomen, she examined my tum very carefully. I had to stand up and sit down, so that she could see where my ample folds of flesh naturally creased and rested. A badly-sighted stoma can cause endless problems, but this nurse knew exactly what she was doing. She carefully marked a small area just to the left of my navel.

"That's where the stoma will be if you need one," she explained.

"Let's hope that I don't, or that it's only temporary." It occurred to me that nothing like this had been done at Casterbridge Hospital even though there had been a slight chance of me needing a stoma back in September 2000. But perhaps, in truth, there hadn't been a slight chance if only a foreign object was going to be removed.

Prof Shaw appeared briefly at lunch time while I was making the best of a glass of water. He appeared happy with how everything was going, and I think he was quite looking forward to getting up to his elbows in my guts. The 31st was going to be a big day for him as well as for me. That afternoon Sally, his nurse, dropped by.

"How are you feeling about things?" she asked anxiously.

"All right," I assured her. "I'm not changing my mind this time if that's what you're wondering. I know having the op is the only option really if I'm going to get better."

"You're very brave."

"Well, I know I'm in good hands. I'm under one of the best surgeons in the country, aren't I?"

"One of the best in the world, actually," she replied.

After my abysmal treatment under Ellman at Casterbridge, I did indeed consider myself fortunate to be in the care of a top surgeon in a highly regarded London teaching hospital. Better care would not be available anywhere in the world. The City and Royal, unlike many a provincial NHS hospital, had an atmosphere of calm professionalism. Most of the time most people knew what they were meant to be doing. The nurses, from many countries, were well trained. Even the ones from agencies stuck to the same ward so that they became part of a well-oiled team.

The 31st of July began early. They had me up at six o'clock for a bath, and then it was one thing after another until I was wheeled off to the theatre at 8.15. It appeared that Prof Shaw was intending to devote most of the day to me. Everything was calm and organised with no unnecessary hanging around, which helped to minimise my understandable anxiety. From the time the anaesthetist got to work, I knew nothing more until I briefly woke up in the recovery room. The next thing I knew I was in intensive care. I had been told to expect up to two days in there after such a big op, so I wasn't surprised. The clock on the wall showed 2pm. I hadn't been told how long the op had been expected to take, as I don't think anyone wanted to hazard a guess, but four or five hours didn't seem that excessive for a thorough job, although it did suggest quite a lot had been done. I gingerly felt my abdomen under the gown. There seemed to be a lot of dressings, but was there also a colostomy bag? I just couldn't tell. Perhaps soon someone would explain to me what had been done. I was surprised at how clear my mind seemed to be after a long anaesthetic.

During the afternoon Dr Baxter appeared at the end of the bed.

"The operation went superbly," he said. I assumed he had been assisting. "We were able to remove virtually all of the mass, but we had to form a stoma."

"Was it cancer?" I managed to croak.

"Some bits looked a bit suspicious. Everything has gone for tests. I'm afraid we won't know for sure for a week or so."

I was getting used to that scenario. Nobody seemed to

know quite how to classify my iffy cells. Before I had time to ask if the colostomy was temporary or permanent, he had disappeared. Perhaps they had removed a bit of my rectum and joined it up again, I thought. I'd just need the stoma for a few weeks while things healed up. Then I'd be back to normal.

Later Mike phoned. It was nice that the call was transferred to the ward and that the nurse was able to bring the phone to my bed. I gave him brief details of the op and explained that pain was controlled by a morphine pump which I could operate myself according to how much I felt I needed. I think he was quite relieved to hear my voice, and learn that things were going reasonably well.

Being in intensive care was extremely boring. I think I was expected to be semi-conscious, but a lot of the time I seemed wide awake with nothing to occupy my thoughts except my medical condition, which I didn't really want to think about, what with all the worrying unknowns. My total intellectual output was telling the nurse my age when she asked, no doubt to test my mental faculties.

"Fifty-seven," I whispered through dry lips.

"You look much younger," she replied. That made me feel quite a lot better.

So long as I lay still, there was no pain. The nurse seemed surprised at how little morphine I was using. Sensory deprivation was my problem. How I longed to be back on the ward with my radio, tapes, books, and magazines. There was absolutely nothing to do in intensive care, and there was too much noise to sleep. There was only one other patient in the small ward, but there seemed to be an awful lot of machinery round both of us which was always beeping and needing attention from the nurses. Unfortunately my earplugs were back in the ward. I tried to amuse myself by working out how many leads and tubes I had attached to me, but gave up.

Late the following morning I was moved back to the ward.

Was I relieved! It seemed I was doing well and that there was absolutely no need for me to stay in intensive care any longer. I managed to reach out to my locker. I slipped my watch on and then found my reading glasses and a magazine. That made me feel a bit more normal.

"Goodness, reading already," a junior doctor remarked as she checked me over. In fact, I wasn't quite so with it as I was pretending to be. It seemed to take half an hour to read a sentence, and when I'd reached the end I'd forgotten the beginning. My brain had turned to jelly. How on earth was I ever going to play chess and Scrabble again?

Next day Mike came up, and stayed about an hour. I didn't feel like talking very much because I still had a tube up my nose and down my throat. It seemed a bit stupid that he had spent eight hours on the return journey to London just to hear a few croaks from me which he could have just as easily have heard over the phone. I couldn't help thinking that hospital visiting was rather a silly ritual. As I looked round the ward, it seemed that after the initial flurry of greetings and the unpacking of clean nighties and bananas etc, most visitors seemed to sit beside their relatives' beds staring into space or reading the papers and magazines they'd brought in for them, and nibbling the grapes.

I continued to make good progress and the following day I sat in a chair for a few hours. The stoma started bubbling slightly and emitting a little fluid into the bag. It showed things were beginning to work as they should. Gradually the various tubes were removed and I was allowed to sip water. By the following Monday the only tube left was a catheter. That afternoon Sally saw me. She had a female colleague with her.

"This is a colleague of mine," she said by way of a vague introduction. I guessed that the woman was a shrink come to secretly assess my mental state after the trauma of losing a body part. I didn't have a lot of time for shrinks because, in general, I didn't think they did much good, sometimes even making things worse. I knew I didn't need one. I was just going to tough things out and get on with life.

"So how are you feeling now?" Sally enquired.

"I think I'm slowly improving. People seem satisfied with my progress."

"You're doing very well," Sally assured me.

"I don't know much about the colostomy," I said. "Has the bowel been joined up, or is it permanent?"

"Are you ready for me to tell you that?" Sally asked with a quick glance at her colleague.

What a stupid question, I thought. If it was bad news why keep me in suspense? It only increased my anxiety.

"As ready as I'll ever be," I replied, trying to be as polite as possible.

"I'm afraid it's permanent."

"Oh! That's rather disappointing seeing Prof told me there was only a twenty per cent chance of that outcome."

"I understand the mass was very firmly attached to the rectum so a section had to be removed. Low down there's not enough to play with to rejoin the ends."

"Yes, Prof did explain that that might be the case. Oh well, I suppose I won't be climbing mountains again."

"You will," Sally replied. "You'll be able to lead a completely normal life once you've recovered. You'll be able to do everything you normally do."

Except shit through the normal orifice, I thought. I looked at her sceptically. "Well, let's hope you're right."

I suspected that she was right, but that I still wouldn't be climbing mountains, not because of the colostomy, but because I was fifty-seven, overweight, and only averagely fit at best. I'd stick to little hills in future. The shrink didn't say anything. She just perched on the edge of the bed looking a bit embarrassed. I suppose she had expected me to break down in floods of tears and start going on about my body image, loss of self-confidence, and all the other crap you're meant to suffer from when you learn you have to go through life with a bag of shit stuck to your tum. I could understand that for a young woman with an attractive body and active sex life, it would indeed be a major trauma, but for a fat old has-been like me... well, the bag would be just another unsightly little bulge to hide under my usual loose shirts and sweaters. If Mike happened to catch the odd glimpse of it, I'd just get the usual 'not a pretty sight', the remark he always made if he caught me in a state of undress. He'd married me for my brain, not my body. I resolved to think of the bag as part of my own anatomy – sort of external plumbing.

Having philosophically accepted my fate, I was now determined to master the physical practicalities of bag management. Because I wasn't allowed to eat, virtually nothing passed into the bag. The stoma wouldn't become active until there was some waste to process. Five days after the operation I was allowed a very light diet consisting of things like yogurt and soup and soon after that the stoma started working. The specialist stoma nurse called once a day and changed the bag for me, encouraging me to gradually start doing it myself. First I had to peel off the existing bag like you would remove a big plaster. Then with a wipe and warm water I had to clean round the stoma, removing all traces of faeces and adhesive from the skin. With another wipe I had to make sure the area was dry so that the new bag would stick well. Then it was just a question of peeling the outer film off the adhesive flange of the new bag, positioning the hole over the stoma, and pressing it down so that it stuck firmly. I would have to do this once or twice a day, depending on my output. I figured that once I was practised and organised, it wouldn't take much longer than normal defecation, the difference being that there was too much to do to read the paper at the same time!

I was quite impressed with the bag technology. It was obvious that the manufacturing company had done years of research. The plastic bag had a soft outer covering which meant it didn't feel clammy against my skin in hot weather. It had a little charcoal filter designed to let out wind without too obvious a smell. You have no control over faeces and wind output because, unlike a normal anus, a stoma has no controlling sphincter muscles. Sometimes the filter didn't work properly because it had become clogged with faeces. If I happened then to be a bit windy, the bag would blow up like a balloon, creating a rather large bulge. However, I soon discovered that there were two sorts of bag, a closed one, and one with a little Velcro-fastened opening. I much preferred the opening sort because it was easy to pop into the loo and release the air if it ballooned, or release the contents down the loo if it was inconvenient to change the bag, for instance when you are out somewhere. I was pleased to learn that I would receive all necessary supplies completely free on the NHS. In fact, my condition was one which entitled me to all medication without prescription charges. All in all, things weren't as bad as I feared they might be.

My second week-end in hospital came along, and the stoma nurse told me she only worked on week-days. I would have to change the bag myself for two days. I panicked a little.

"The nurses will help you if you can't manage," she said.

But I was determined to manage by myself, and I did. After all, it was hardly rocket science.

The stoma wasn't a great problem – the heat was. Early August 2003 had the highest temperature ever recorded in London. Everyone sweltered, and it was amazing that the nurses remained so calm in such trying conditions. Ironically, it was the agency nurse from Australia who complained the most. "All our hospitals are air-conditioned," she explained. Well, they would be, I thought. Temperatures of 35 degrees Celsius plus are the norm in Australia, whereas they virtually never occur in London. I lay on my bed in thin cotton pyjamas and sweated all the time. As I wasn't allowed to eat for five days, it was like starving in a sauna. The weight just fell off me. The skin on my arms and legs looked crepy and saggy, my boobs and buttocks practically disappeared, and when I got home and weighed myself, I was down to ten stone. For about the first time in my life I was the correct weight for my height, yet I felt and looked terrible. I quickly decided I didn't do thin, and I didn't feel normal again until I'd put on a stone. Hospitals are particularly uncomfortable in hot weather because for reasons of hygiene, everything is covered in plastic. To make life bearable, I draped a double thickness of towel over my plastic-covered pillow, and lay on top of the cotton blankets. Just a sheet between me and the plastic-covered mattress wasn't enough. The nurses seemed quite pleased; they never had to change my bed because I never got into it.

Mike timed his next visit to coincide with the peak of the heat wave. I'd warned him on the phone that London was a furnace compared to the south coast with its moderating sea breezes, and that he was to wear the minimum necessary for decency. He arrived red-faced in a sweat-stained shirt and seemed absolutely exhausted. We decided that he shouldn't come again. After all, we talked on the phone every evening, and if I desperately needed anything he could post it.

Once I was a bit more mobile, I sometimes sought relief from the heat and stuffiness of the ward by sitting out on the fire escape. I was five storeys up where the sultry air was marginally fresher than at street level. Then they stopped us going out there. I suppose they thought we might start jumping off it, a distinct possibility seeing many patients on the ward had cancer.

A week after the operation Prof Shaw put in an appearance. He seemed very pleased with my progress, but rather apologetic that a permanent colostomy had been necessary.

"If I had been able to operate a year sooner, the outcome would have almost certainly been much better," he explained.

A year sooner, I thought, not two or three years. But

according to my dubious medical history, the lump had been there in a relatively unchanged condition since it was detected in the scan done in August 2000. However, my own symptoms suggested it hadn't started forming until the early summer of 2002. His remark pretty well confirmed my own scenario, that the lump, whatever it was, was removed in September 2000, but that then something else formed. However, I knew it was pointless trying to turn my case back to the 'foreign object' scenario. It was better to use Prof's remark to strengthen the negligent follow-up care scenario. I reached for my writing pad and wrote a note to Bentham. After mentioning the outcome of the operation, and Prof Shaw's remark, I wrote: 'It seems that if Ellman at Casterbridge Hospital had had the humility to refer me to Prof Shaw in September 2000 after he claimed he could not remove the mass, my chances of being treated completely successfully would have been high. I simply cannot understand why I was not referred to a centre of excellence as I am a relatively young person with no other health problems. The lies I was told about my condition lulled me into a false sense of security so that I was not inclined to ask for a second opinion or referral to another surgeon. The course of action taken by Ellman seems inexplicable.'

It seemed to me that I now had a rock-solid case for negligence even though, in my opinion, it was based entirely on a cover-up scenario rather than the truth. The fact that I now had a permanent disability would mean that the damages would rocket. What I had originally thought might be a few thousand for an unnecessary operation to remove a foreign object, could now even reach six figures. What would I do with £100,000 I wondered? I didn't really need it, and I'd far rather have the truth about my medical condition. However, it seemed increasingly likely that although I'd get a tidy sum of money, I'd never get the truth.

Thirteen days after the operation the doctors decided that as I had made an excellent recovery, I could go home. But first I had to be told the result of the pathology tests. Dr Baxter and Sally came to see me. The fact that Sally was with him suggested it was bad news.

"We have the results from the path lab," Dr Baxter said. "I'm afraid they did find borderline malignancy in some cells. But the good news is there is no sign of spread beyond the mass we removed. But to be sure, I think it would be a good idea for you to have a course of chemotherapy."

It was yet another blow, just when I thought I was doing well.

"It's one thing after another," I said. Sometimes everything did become too much, and I could feel the tears welling up. Sally took over.

"Would you like to phone your husband?" she asked.

"Yes, I would please."

"I'll take you to Sister's office. You can have some privacy in there."

This was the sort of consideration that seemed to be the norm at the City and Royal. Fortunately Mike was in and answered quickly.

"First the good news," I said. "I'm coming home this afternoon. Now the bad news. They found some cancer cells. They don't think it's much. But I've got to have chemo."

"Oh dear. But I suppose it wasn't entirely unexpected. It could be worse, I suppose."

As I would have expected, Mike was trying to be optimistic. But there was good reason for optimism. As Prof Shaw had always suspected, mine seemed to be a semi-dormant type of cancer. For all I knew, it had remained much as it had been in 1981. It certainly wasn't going to kill me in the next few weeks, or even the next few years for that matter. Modern chemo might completely knock it out. I tried to look on the bright side. The worst thought was that I might temporarily lose my hair. Why were we women so fixated on our hair? Prof Shaw was nearly bald yet still managed to be dead sexy.

The young women doctors in his entourage all seemed to blush when he spoke to them, and I wasn't totally immune to his charms myself. Then there was the legal aspect to think about. It was reasonable to conclude that the cancer would not have developed had I had proper treatment when I needed it back in 2000. One small step for the cancer, one giant leap for the damages, I thought. But what's wealth if you haven't got health? Give me the latter any day. The thought of the rocketing damages was only a thin coating of sugar on a bitter pill.

CHAPTER 21

It was lovely to be home again. I had to take things easy, so I spent quite a lot of time on my lounger in the shade of the garden with Mike bringing out a steady supply of chilled fruit juice. Life could be worse. The heat continued, but as we were only a few miles from the coast, it was never too intense. The local stoma nurse called once a week to check that I was managing things OK. In the main, I was, and it was a great relief not to be rushing to the loo every hour or so as I had been.

For a while housework was out of the question, so I got a cleaning lady. Mike did the shopping, but as I got stronger I went with him, just about managing to pick things off the shelves while he guided the trolley and did all the lifting. Due to the heat, the garden didn't need much attention, but I knew I would need a gardener to tidy up in the autumn. With Mike's help I cooked my usual simple meals, and I was soon able to do a few light tasks like picking the plums from the low branches of our tree. Life rapidly changed for the better about three and a half weeks after the op when I started driving short distances.

I had to go to the City and Royal for a check-up on the 27th of August. I was determined to get myself fit enough to cope with the tube and the walks between the coach station and the tube station, and on to the hospital. It was just a question of slowly building up my physical activity. At first I walked for five minutes – just to the end of the close and back. After a few days I was doing half a mile in ten minutes. Then I gradually worked up to a mile in twenty minutes, doing this without pain or tiredness. I knew then that I was up to coping with most normal everyday activities. The trip to the City and Royal was a doddle, and the junior doctor who checked me over seemed most impressed by my rapid recovery.

Now that I was over the op, the chemotherapy had to be arranged.

"You'll be able to have it at Casterbridge," the doctor explained.

"I don't think that would be a very good idea," I replied. "You see, I'm currently suing that hospital. Couldn't it be done at Sandcliffe? That's only seven miles away. Obviously, I don't want to have to come up here for it. The travelling would be a bit much if I wasn't feeling well after the treatment."

"I'll have to make enquiries," she said. "I can understand your concern, but it would really be best if you had your treatment at Casterbridge."

"But I'll be under a consultant who has already told me that chemo won't be effective, and who has basically already written me off."

The doctor looked amazed but didn't say anything. She obviously knew nothing about my recent history, and I wasn't going into it. Everything was left undecided, although I had a horrible suspicion that I was going to be pushed back to Casterbridge Hospital. I thought about it all on the long journey home. No way was I going back to Casterbridge. Next day I sent a fax to Sally making my views quite clear. I knew I had the right to choose where I had my treatment.

A week later Sally phoned me. She explained that Sand-cliffe Hospital didn't do chemo, and that if I didn't want it done at Casterbridge, I would have to go to Titchmouth Hospital. I was perfectly agreeable to that. Titchmouth was only a forty-five minute drive along the coast, so it would be considerably easier than trailing up to London. I asked her to put the wheels in motion.

Ten days later I had an appointment with consultant oncologist Dr Karen Grant. She was young and glamorous with an amazing shock of golden curly hair.

"Hi, I'm Karen Grant," she greeted me. She seemed very warm and friendly. "So, you've been under Prof Shaw up at the City and Royal. He's written me a very full account of what's been done, and the pathology findings. Who's the lucky one, then? He's an amazingly skilled surgeon, you know."

"Yes, I've had very good treatment," I assured her.

"I studied under him. He's so clever, and not only that, he's such a, -er, such a nice man."

I smiled at her. 'Nice'! Perhaps she meant to say 'gorgeous hunk' or 'sex god'. She was smiling too. We were like two teenagers sharing a passion for some pop idol.

"I've not seen him for over a year," she went on rather wistfully. I smirked, as she would have known I'd had regular face-to-face contact with him for some months. I felt that Karen Grant and I would get on very well. She'd be particularly interested in me, as I would give her an excuse to write 'Dear Julian' letters about my progress even if they weren't strictly necessary.

We then got down to the serious matter of my chemotherapy.

"There's a number of things we could do," Dr Grant explained. "You can have a combination of drugs. That would be quite strong treatment – not very pleasant, and your hair would fall out. Or you could just have carboplatin by itself. The side effects from that are minimal, and it's generally very effective. Or we can do nothing – just observe you closely and do something if things start going down hill."

She'd put it quite clearly, but I didn't really feel I was capable of judging what would be best. I've always been a bit of a middle-of-the road type of person, so the middle course seemed the right one.

"I think at this stage I'll just have the carboplatin," I said. "That way the stronger treatment can be kept in case it becomes necessary later. I'm not sure I'd be happy not having any treatment. If the cancer got a hold again, I'd think that if I'd had treatment I'd have been OK."

"That's fine."

I think Dr Grant herself would have recommended the carboplatin if I had left it to her.

"You'll be able to start your treatment next week. You'll have six courses at three week intervals, and except for a day or two after each session, it shouldn't affect you at all."

I started my chemo at the end of September. Mike came to Titchmouth with me, as I was not sure whether I would be fit to drive home after the treatment. It was a long drawn-out affair. First I had to see the registrar, have a blood test, and be weighed and measured for height. This was all so that the correct concentration of drug could be mixed. There was then a long wait while the lab supplied the right infusion. Then in the early afternoon I was called for treatment. I was given anti-sickness pills and then, after immersing my hand in a bowl of warm water to make the veins stand up, a canula was put in the back of my hand through which the drug was delivered. It took about one and a half hours to drip in, but I was lucky. Some people were tied to their drips for four or five hours. It was a good job we all had comfy reclining armchairs to sit in and plenty of magazines. I looked around at my fellow patients and played 'spot the wig', which in most cases wasn't too difficult. Some people preferred a headscarf, while baseball caps were popular with younger women. Many, of course, like me, did not have hair loss. Most people looked rather weak and ill. I felt fine, and I think compared with other patients I looked positively robust. Somehow I didn't feel I was in the right place. Did I really need this unpleasant and potentially harmful treatment? Was it really necessary?

I still felt fine after the treatment and drove home. I

regarded Mike as a lousy driver, so much preferred to drive myself. At teatime I felt really hungry, and ended up stuffing my face most of the evening. I later learnt that this was the effect of the steroids in the anti-sickness medication. I had been given more anti-sickness pills to take, but hadn't used them. Then, at about 11.30pm just as I was off to bed, the sickness kicked in. I was throwing up all night. But by the morning I was OK again, so I just took it easy for the next day or two. I took the anti-sickness pills but they made me feel strangely agitated. I thought enduring a few hours of sickness was preferable.

Legal matters had gone very quiet. Mr Bentham was trying to arrange a case management conference at Jeremy Carr's chambers in London. Finding a date when Carr, Bentham, Dr Jessop, the independent expert, and ourselves were all going to be available was quite a problem. Eventually it was fixed for the afternoon of the 9th of October. The idea was that we would all be able to discuss the case together and it was hoped that Mr Jessop could be persuaded to strengthen certain aspects of his report so that negligence in the treatment of my condition could be shown. As mine was a civil action, firm proof was not essential. Balance of probability was good enough, and I felt that a little tweaking here and there in Jessop's report was all that was needed.

The day of the conference arrived. Mike and I took the coach to London while Bentham went up by train. Carr's chambers were somewhere deep in the Inns of Court. Mike had visited the area a few times when he had been in practice and reckoned he knew his way around, so I meekly followed him, having myself never been anywhere near that part of London. We turned down a little alleyway off the Strand and entered a secluded area of gracious old buildings round little courtyards. People in black gowns bustled about carrying files tied up with red tape. The atmosphere reminded me of the quadrangle of an Oxbridge college, and it all seemed far removed from the frantic commercial activity of the London streets. With some difficulty we found Carr's chambers. Beside the doorway there was a long list of all the barristers who practised there. We entered, and were shown to a slightly shabby waiting area with ancient leather sofas. It all had a rather junior common room feeling. A few minutes later Bentham joined us, and then Mr Jessop appeared. We sat around talking about everything except the case while waiting to be called to Carr's room. I wondered what Jeremy Carr would be like. I didn't know any barristers but I assumed they were mostly pedantic old fuddy-duddies whose brains had atrophied under the weight and warmth of their wigs. Then a figure appeared further along the hall we were sitting in, and then disappeared into another room.

"That was Jeremy Carr," Bentham whispered to me. I had just caught a glimpse of a dark and handsome man who didn't look a day over forty. In other words Jeremy Carr seemed very OK.

Eventually we were shown into his consulting room where we all sat round a shiny mahogany table with all the necessary files in front of us. The walls were lined with serious-looking leather-bound tomes with gilt lettering. Carr took control of the proceedings. I was immediately impressed by him – the dark good looks, the rather unruly hair and boyish charm, the deep, well modulated but not over-posh voice, and perhaps most important of all, the razor-sharp mind. I had always regarded myself as pretty much on the ball, but in the presence of Carr I felt very second league, although my complete ignorance of the working of the law probably had something to do with it. Bentham also seemed rather awe-struck. He and Carr had worked together before, and Bentham had already told me that he thought Carr was an exceptionally good barrister. Bentham assumed the role of a submissive secretary, listening carefully, making copious notes, and occasionally directing Carr to various sections of all the files.

Jessop sat with his arms folded, looking rather sulky. I had the feeling he didn't want to be there. Mike was ready with a yellow legal pad in front of him to make notes on anything he felt was important. I just had my file of medical notes and Jessop's report ready for referring to. Although, as the plaintiff, I was in some ways the most important person there, I felt very much at the bottom of the pecking order. I really didn't know what was going to happen, and I was already worrying about how much it was all costing me.

Carr wasted no time in closely questioning Jessop about aspects of his report. In every case where Jessop had used phrases such as 'not best practice', or had suggested that something might have been done differently, or where something had not been done which should have been, Carr asked him if it could possibly be regarded as negligence or professional misconduct. The guiding principle seemed to be whether Ellman had acted as most consultant gynaecologists would have done in a similar situation. On every point raised Jessop was adamant that he could not change the wording of his report. Even when he conceded that he himself would have done something differently, he would not agree that how Ellman had gone about things amounted to negligence. He also kept raising the point that whatever had been done or not done, the outcome would have been the same for me. In other words, he seemed to assume that even back in 2000 I was a pretty hopeless case, and it was inevitable that I would develop cancer and lose my rectum.

I began to think that his attitude was totally unreasonable. In the back of my mind were thoughts about his relationship with Professor Shaw. I wondered whether his number one priority was to ensure that his close colleague was protected. Yet I felt that this could be misplaced loyalty because, as far as I was concerned, Prof Shaw had done absolutely nothing wrong and there was no way he was ever going to be drawn into the action. Or had I just succumbed to the great professor's charm and authority? I didn't think so. At very worst, he might have been economical with the truth. Sometimes I felt he knew exactly what had been going on, but would never tell me. I didn't expect him to; doctors just didn't tell tales on each other.

The conference went on and on. Carr asked the questions, Jessop answered them, I clarified various points about what happened when, and how I remembered things, Mike and Bentham made notes. In the end Carr turned to me.

"Well, Mrs Bland, it seems from what Mr Jessop has been saying that your case is very weak. I think you've already accepted that it would be impossible to prove your 'foreign object' theory, and it seems that although in some respects your treatment was not of a good standard, it's simply not possible to show that anything specific has directly caused your current condition. I can only reiterate what I have already advised you – you would be throwing good money after bad to pursue matters any further."

I felt utterly drained. Mr Jessop looked smug, and Mike looked confused. Bentham scribbled away on his pad. I really didn't know what to say, so I voiced the first thing that came into my head.

"But what about the forged histology report? That is evidence of wrong-doing. Couldn't it be used as a sort of way in, a way of casting doubt on other things?" I felt I wasn't expressing myself very well. Jessop looked rather alarmed. For his report he had been asked to comment on the nature of the fabricated histology report and the unusual handwritten back-up documentation, and he had conceded that it all seemed rather irregular, but had left it at that. Carr had not questioned him on that part of his report. I went on.

"The name 'Appleyard' on the recently typed report doesn't appear anywhere in the handwritten documents. Someone, Ellman I suspect, just plucked it from the air, it seems. Appleyard wasn't a consultant in 1981 – I've proved that."

"It would indeed be an embarrassing point," Carr replied. "But how could it be used to help your case? It's very peripheral – it wouldn't progress matters."

I could understand Carr's attitude, but I didn't share it. As a barrister, he was only interested in winning my case and obtaining a large sum of damages for me. I was more interested in truth and justice. So long as I did not end up out of pocket, I was not over-concerned about money. I wanted to find out exactly what had been going on, and I wanted Ellman suitably disciplined, preferably struck off.

Mike was looking at me. I knew he wanted me to admit defeat. It did seem to be the end of the road. Carr spoke again.

"Mrs Bland, I feel I must warn you that if you continue to pursue this case, your costs could rise to £100,000. The costs on the other side would be similar. If you then ultimately lost, you would have to meet both sides' costs."

"Yes, I know. It would wipe me out financially. We could even lose the house." I couldn't risk it. I'd lost my rectum and my good health, but I did still have good financial security. I wasn't going to risk losing that as well.

"You see," Carr went on, "the other side could claim that because you chose to stop seeing Mr Ellman, you're the author of your own misfortune. I'm sorry to have to be the devil's advocate as it were, but I must make clear the risk you face if you continue to pursue this case."

"Yes, I know," I said once more. "I'll have to end it. I can't risk going on."

I think I heard a sigh of relief from Mike but, somewhat surprisingly, both Carr and Bentham looked rather deflated. Well, I suppose they would. The gravy train had hit the buffers. It would have been to their financial advantage for me to have gone on, bearing in mind that the fees they were earning from the case would probably amount to nearly as much as my damages. Had they secretly hoped I would carry on? Had all the dire warnings just been so that they could claim they had given me best advice if things had gone wrong?

Carr and Bentham were looking at each other. They seemed to read each other well. I knew they had worked together before, possibly on the case involving a certain Emma Bentham. They both knew that Ellman was a rogue, and I think they both thought I did have a case, although it was going to be virtually impossible to prove. A strange silence fell around the table. Carr was looking at a section of my medical notes. At last he spoke.

"I think this case may still be alive," he said cautiously. "Perhaps we should consider the role played by Mrs Bland's GP, er, Dr Foyle."

"I suspect he always knew what had been going on," I said. "But I've never thought to drag him into it because he's not the main culprit. It would only have complicated matters."

"I think, though," Carr went on, "we have evidence for breach of duty on his part. I'm looking at the two letters Mr Ellman wrote to Dr Foyle towards the end of March 2001 once he knew Mrs Bland had reported him to the GMC and that therefore the professional relationship had broken down."

We all flipped through our copies of my notes until we found the letters. Carr read the second one.

"'Unfortunately your patient failed to arrive in the clinic today for her planned re-appointment. However, in the light of the recent communications, I suspect that she is more inclined to seek her care elsewhere and in addition I am not entirely sure that I would be inclined to disagree with that sentiment. May I therefore leave it up to you to rearrange.'"

Carr glanced up at us all. "I think this letter makes it quite clear that both Mrs Bland and Mr Ellman have accepted that at this time the professional relationship has ended. It also seems that Mr Ellman now considers it is the duty of Dr Foyle to arrange her future care. Mr Jessop, as a consultant yourself, perhaps you could help us on the matter. I suppose it does occasionally happen that problems occur between a consultant and a patient. Could you enlighten us on any laid-down procedure in such a situation?"

Mr Jessop looked slightly alarmed. The case had taken an unexpected turn. "Yes, there are guidelines," he replied. "And Mr Ellman followed them correctly. He informed the patient's GP of the situation. It was then up to the GP to refer the patient to another consultant."

"Could Mrs Bland have referred herself to another consultant?"

"No. All referrals are done via the GP. The GP is the conduit between the patient and the consultant."

"I see." Carr's close questioning of Jessop went on. Bentham was scribbling away like mad and looking very intent. They were on the scent again, like a couple of bloodhounds. "Is it reasonable to expect that Mrs Bland should know that she should now see her GP? There doesn't appear to be any letter instructing her to do so."

"Unless a patient had been in a similar situation before, they probably wouldn't know they had to go back to their GP," Jessop conceded. "But most people would see their GP because they might need on-going treatment."

"But that didn't apply in Mrs Bland's case. She believed she was completely well in early 2001. She wasn't receiving any treatment. Dr Foyle should have known that. Was it reasonable to expect that she would contact him, or should he have been pro-active?"

I really felt we were getting somewhere now. Jessop was looking very uncomfortable.

"In my opinion, it would have been better if the GP had made contact with Mrs Bland," he said cautiously. "But the GP knows their patients. There may have been a good reason why he chose not to."

I believe there was a very good reason, I thought to myself. I was meant to have a lump in me which didn't exist. How would that be explained to a new consultant? It was better to do nothing. I probably wouldn't have been referred to a new consultant even if I had gone to the GP.

Carr kept up the grilling.

"So the GP could have phoned Mrs Bland, or written to her, inviting her to come in and discuss the situation."

"He could have."

"But should he have done so, given his knowledge of Mrs Bland's health?"

"It would have been best practice."

"So what does he do? Let's see." Carr directed us to another section of my notes. "He just writes, 'See letter from Mr Ellman'."

"That would be so that if Mrs Bland came in and saw one of his partners, they would raise the matter," Jessop explained.

"But then Mrs Bland had no further contact with the surgery for just over a year when she attended with a respiratory infection. Records indicate that Mrs Bland is not popping into the surgery every week or two - it's more like every year or two, if that."

Jessop couldn't think of anything to say and sat looking sulky. Carr and Bentham were looking at each other again.

"Well, it does seem to me there may be a case of breach of duty against Dr Foyle," Carr went on. "The letters from Ellman, and the notes made by Dr Foyle provide good evidence. I'm not at all sure how the GP's non-action could be defended. Mr Jessop, would you be willing to write a short report on Dr Foyle's handling of this matter, concentrating particularly on what he should have done on receipt of Mr Ellman's letters?"

"Yes, I can do that," Jessop replied, without enthusiasm I thought.

At this point I remembered something else about the letters to which I thought I should draw Carr's attention.

"If you look at the first letter Ellman wrote," I said, "you will see he says he will phone Foyle to discuss things. If that call was made, there should be something in my notes about it as it might have contained information about my condition. I don't think the call was ever made, but if it was, it told Foyle something about me that for some reason couldn't be written in my notes. Perhaps Mr Jessop would like to comment on that as well in his report."

Carr took this up. "If a GP discusses a patient with a consultant on the phone, is it normally noted down?"

"It should be," Jessop confirmed. "But remember how busy GPs often are. There are bound to be oversights."

Bentham was still scribbling away, but now looked up from his pad. "Mr Jessop, I'll write to you with specific instructions as to what to include in your report about Dr Foyle. Will you be able to deal with it fairly quickly?"

"Within a month. I'm afraid I've got to go now – another appointment." He stood up and picked up his briefcase. Good, I thought, one less ridiculous hourly rate to finance. These top professionals sitting around me were charging per hour what most ordinary mortals took a week to earn. I tried to keep it firmly in the back of my mind that I was paying for this whole caboodle. It was all going on for longer than I had anticipated, and I reckoned it had already reached the cost of a world cruise.

The possible case against Dr Foyle was discussed further after Jessop's departure. It was agreed that I should think the matter over before giving instructions. I made it clear that my strong inclination was to go for Foyle. I knew that I had now lost something over £13,000 in legal costs so far, and I wanted to get it back, plus a bit more. The question was, would I get it back even if I was successful?

"What sort of damages might I get if it can be shown that Foyle's lack of action has probably caused my present condition?" I asked.

"Mm. Permanent colostomy," said Carr, reaching into his briefcase for a little booklet.

How could anyone place a monetary value on a human rectum, I wondered. What was the worth of the ability to have a conventional shit? It all seemed so surreal.

"Colostomy – permanent," Carr read out. "£77,000, and these figures are soon to be updated."

"Goodness me!" I exclaimed. "That's a lot. It's hardly like losing a limb, you know."

"But that figure is for a young person," Carr added. "Anything you would get would be reduced on account of your age. But you'd still get perhaps £40 to £50,000."

"And what about the cancer aspect?"

"Very difficult to quantify. If, unfortunately, it is incurable and your expected lifespan is short, then we could be doubling that figure. If it's easily curable we'd perhaps be looking at another £10,000. It's a difficult area."

"So it's worth going on," I concluded. "There would still be plenty over even after I've deducted the costs of the case against Ellman which I know I can't recover."

"Financially it would be worthwhile to continue," Carr agreed. "But you must ask yourself if you want the stress. You may have to appear in court. The case seems quite good, but I would anticipate that the other side will put up a strong defence. Do you want this strain if you're not too well?"

"I'll let Mr Bentham know in a day or two," I said.

After three and a half hours the conference ended. I was exhausted. It had taken an unexpected and dramatic turn. As one door had closed, another had opened. We just managed to catch the six o'clock coach. Soon we were stuck in the rush hour traffic around Hammersmith. I knew that once we were cruising down the motorway we'd both fall asleep, so I talked things over with Mike there and then.

"I am going to sue Foyle," I said emphatically. "I've known from the beginning he's been covering up for Ellman. Look how he didn't refer me back to the hospital when I had those bowel problems after the February 2000 op. He's always known exactly what's been going on. So when I stopped seeing Ellman he didn't try to refer me to someone new because he knew damn well I didn't really need referring. I was OK at that time. It was just unfortunate for them, and me, that I developed another lump of some kind. Foyle will have to defend himself. Perhaps this will be a sort of new way to the truth. Perhaps Foyle will spill the beans."

"You'll have to find yourself a new doctor," Mike muttered before nodding off.

CHAPTER 22

The very next day I gave Bentham written instructions that I now wished to bring proceedings against Dr Foyle. My letter to him was quite long, as I wanted to make it clear that Foyle should have been well aware for some months that I was dissatisfied with my poor treatment under Ellman. It therefore should have been quite obvious to him that he had to take control of the situation. Ellman had mentioned in an earlier letter that I appeared rather confused about my condition, which should have alerted Foyle to the possibility that I would not realise the potential seriousness of my problems and therefore seek help myself. In my mind it all added up to a quite obvious breach of duty. I also pointed out that Mike and I had been with Foyle and his partners for over twenty years. It was a well-run practice, and we had both been perfectly satisfied with the care we had received until this incident. The negligence therefore seemed inexplicable, but I added that I had my own dark thoughts on the matter.

During the next few weeks nothing much happened as we were waiting for the report on Foyle from Jessop, who seemed to be dragging his feet. The report we required seemed relatively straightforward to me, so I could not understand why it was taking so long to produce.

Meanwhile I carried on with my chemo. I had a dose every three weeks. As the medication had no immediate effect on me, I was able to drive myself up to Titchmouth and back. Then I'd stuff myself all evening and throw up all night. After that I was fine again. Whatever it was they gave me to control the side-effects while I was receiving the chemo made me agitated and aggressive. Driving home along the motorway I'd find myself doing ninety in the outside lane along with all the stressed reps and boy racers. I'd be fantasising about what I'd like to do to Ellman's car one dark night. Would my vegetable knife be up to slashing the tyres? Orange paint would look good splashed over the bodywork. For some unfathomable reason I imagined that Ellman drove a dark blue BMW. In fact, I hadn't a clue what he drove. Anyway orange paint would look good on shiny dark blue. While I was about it, I'd also attack Foyle's car. I didn't know what he drove either, although I had once seen him in an ancient Metro, which was more likely to have been the wife's runabout, or the sprog's old banger. I'd spread baked beans all over the bonnet, as a hint to him to spill the beans. I was still hoping that somehow the case would swing back to Ellman, as he was the real culprit. Foyle was just his sidekick. Fortunately all these fantasies remained just that. I knew full well that I had to stay squeaky clean and pursue my grievances through the proper legal channels.

I saw Dr Karen Grant (or Goldilocks as I called her) before my treatments. After the usual brief meeting of the Titchmouth branch of the Prof Shaw appreciation society, i.e. had either of us seen or heard from the great man, we discussed my condition. Everything appeared to be going well. She assured me that my CA125 readings were falling, although she didn't tell me the actual values. She felt my tum and seemed satisfied. Then I'd wait while the lab mixed up the evil brew to be infused into me. The nurses would call me after some hours and fix up the drip. As the treatments went on I got the vague impression that the nurses' attitude to me was slightly offhand, nothing that you could complain about, but not quite as attentive and sympathetic as that received by the other patients. I always seemed to be the last one called from the waiting area, despite the fact that I was receiving one of the simplest infusions. When the treatment had finished, I'd often be left hooked up to the empty bags. If I drew the matter to their attention, I'd be left even longer. I got the strange feeling that the nurses thought I shouldn't be there. The problem was, I shared their thoughts. Did I really need this chemotherapy?

I suffered a minor setback in early November. I returned to Sandcliffe Hospital to have the stents removed from my ureters. They were no longer necessary because the mass blocking them had been removed. The minor operation went smoothly, and I was able to pee perfectly normally afterwards. But when I got home I developed a high temperature. As I was on chemo it was taken seriously. I was admitted, horror of horrors, into Casterbridge Hospital, but fortunately was soon transferred to Sandcliffe when it was found the stent operation had caused a kidney infection. I was put on intravenous antibiotics and recovered after a few days.

Another shock to the system was having to pay the bill for the case conference. It came to £5,691, which, as I had calculated, would have paid for a world cruise at the bottom end of the market. However, my view was that if it ultimately led to a successful action against Foyle, it would have been worth it. And speaking of cruises, it was around this time that I read in the Casterbridge Clarion that the lucky couple Emma and Joseph Bentham had won the paper's competition for a cruise on the brand new Queen Mary II. Money goes where money is was my initial thought. What about all those people on the council estates struggling to make ends meet who must have entered the competition? Why did a stinking rich solicitor have to win it? Then my eyes really came out on stalks. Emma Bentham! The woman who had won the court action against Ellman. She *was* his wife! No wonder Bentham seemed so interested in my case.

By the middle of December Dr Jessop had still not produced what was assumed to be a short and simple report, although it had been expected in early November. To me, the delay seemed inexcusable. As the suspected negligence had taken place in March 2001, it was going to be necessary to get a court summons by March 2004 if I wasn't to be time-barred. Once more time seemed to be running out. Jessop had also recommended that Bentham should obtain another report from an independent expert qualified to comment specifically on GPs. Once again I had the feeling that for some reason Jessop didn't want to provide a report. Why didn't he just say so? Anyway, Bentham duly lined up a Dr Anthony Read who appeared to have had considerable experience in medical litigation against GPs.

We finally got Jessop's report at the end of January along with his bill for £900. My heart sank as I read it. He had gone right back to the beginning of my troubles in December 1999. He concluded that Foyle had provided excellent care in fast-tracking me to a consultant gynaecologist at that point, and I fully agreed with him. He then followed my care through all the visits I had made with my bowel problems, and again concluded that I had received perfectly satisfactory care. Somehow he then jumped straight to August 2002 when I returned with bowel problems and saw Dr Wilson who also fast-tracked me to a gynaecologist. That was also good practice, Jessop concluded, and I could not disagree. The big problem was that the report totally ignored the one issue that Bentham had instructed him to address – Foyle's non-action on receiving letters from Ellman indicating that the professional relationship between us had broken down, but making clear that I needed on-going care. The report was utterly useless because it appeared that Jessop had deliberately not followed the instructions given to him. No way was I going to pay his £900 fee.

Almost boiling over with rage, I sat down at my word processor and banged out a long letter to Bentham pointing out all the above. I concluded that unless Jessop was willing to substantially alter his report, and include the verbal comments he had made at the conference about the GP's responsibility, he should not be paid. I hoped that Bentham would back me on this point.

A few days later we discussed the matter on the phone. It turned out that Bentham was as surprised and outraged as I was. He had sent the report to Jeremy Carr for his comments, and was in full agreement that Jessop should not be paid his fee.

"I'll never use him again," he said. "I've never experienced anything like this before."

It was agreed that we should now go ahead immediately and request a report from Dr Anthony Read, as time was now getting short. In fact, during the following month there was no progress as Bentham was very involved in other cases. Eventually I had to write to him to remind him that we had to issue a summons against Foyle by the beginning of April.

Meanwhile my course of chemotherapy ended, thank goodness. I had a scan which showed some scar tissue which I was told must be regularly monitored. My CA125 blood test gave a reading of seven on a scale where zero to thirty was regarded as normal. I interpreted all this as indicating that I did not now have cancer, although I accepted that frequent checks would be necessary for some time.

Goldilocks seemed delighted with my progress.

"Prof Shaw must have done a good job," she commented. "I'm sure he removed all cancerous and potentially cancerous material. He's so thorough, you know." No praise was high enough for her idol, but I found myself in full agreement with her.

"I think I'm quite fortunate," I replied, "but there is something I find very confusing. In October 2002 at Casterbridge, I was told my cancer was inoperable and untreatable by chemotherapy. In other words it seemed likely to be terminal. Now, as far as we can tell, I've had a successful operation, and successful chemo. Why do you think I was given such a bad prognosis?"

Goldilocks's cheerful demeanour seemed to evaporate. Just how much did she know? Had she been having secret little phone conversations with 'dear Julian'? She recovered quickly, but I could sense that her brain was in overdrive.

"I would suggest that your oncologist at Casterbridge hadn't given sufficient consideration to the twenty-year time gap since your previous cancer diagnosis. I believe he thought you had an on-going condition."

I didn't comment but I immediately wondered if Oswald had been mislead by the fabricated histology report, which, of course, had a contemporary look to it. I kept on wondering about a lot of things, and I knew I would never be able to put it all behind me and move on, as they say. All I could hope for was that Foyle, in trying to defend himself, would spill the beans. However, I was still waiting for the report from Dr Read to see whether it was going to be worth taking action against Foyle. Everything seemed to be moving so slowly.

The draft report finally arrived in late March. It was exactly what we wanted. It included everything we had asked Jessop to comment upon, and which he had completely ignored. Put briefly, Dr Read's conclusion was that it was irresponsible for Foyle to have done nothing about arranging my future care under a new consultant. He should have made arrangements for me to have seen another consultant at Casterbridge, or, preferably, outside the area. Before doing anything he should have contacted me by letter or phone so that we could have discussed the situation. He should not have relied on the possibility of me appearing at the surgery myself. The only area in which he was more circumspect was the likely effect that the lack of supervision would have had on my condition, although he was prepared to suggest that regular monitoring would have enabled me to have surgery earlier with a more satisfactory outcome.

On the strength of this report, Bentham immediately issued a claim against Foyle in the Casterbridge County Court. We were up and running again. I wasted no time in moving to another medical practice. I thought Mike should move too, but he was so happy with the way Dr Wilson looked after his diabetes that he decided to stay.

I suggested to Bentham that by far the best person to comment on the likely outcome of having further surgery sooner than I had done was Prof Shaw, the only person other than Ellman who had intimate hands-on knowledge of my innards. Bentham therefore wrote to him asking if he would be willing to write a report detailing how the delay might have affected my condidtion, and including a prognosis for my future health. He made it quite clear that no action was contemplated against the City and Royal, or against Shaw himself.

I was not surprised when I heard that Prof Shaw was not willing to produce such a report. He pointed out that I was still partially under his care and that it would therefore be inappropriate for him to be involved in my legal case. However, as I would have expected, he was helpful, and recommended that a report was obtained from Mr Jonathan Muir, a gynaecologist in Titchmouth. Bentham was quickly in communication with Muir, and was informed that a report could be produced within six weeks.

While all this was going on, Mike decided to pursue a different avenue. He had always been particularly aggrieved by the gloomy prognosis given to us by Dr Oswald at Casterbridge in October 2002. At that time he had predicted that surgery was likely to be unsuccessful, and chemotherapy or radiotherapy ineffective. Now, eighteen months later, I had had both successful surgery and chemotherapy and, so far as it was possible to tell, I was free of cancer. Had we not pushed very hard for referral to the City and Royal, I would possibly now be dead. I think Mike had been very much more upset by the prognosis than I had been because he actually believed Oswald, whereas I had suspected all along that he had been fed false information by Ellman and that things weren't quite as bad as they had seemed. Anyway, Mike wanted to see what Oswald had to say for himself. In his defence, would he let slip something about Ellman? It was possible. Like me, Mike suspected that in going for Foyle we were suing the wrong person, and that if anything could be done to turn the case back on to Ellman, it should be attempted.

Mike's letter to the Chief Executive simply asked how Dr Oswald justified his prognosis which subsequent events had shown to be wide of the mark. About three weeks later, once Dr Oswald had had a chance to review my notes, we received a reply. Basically, it was a very brief whitewash. It appeared that Oswald had concluded that my disease was extensive, but seemed to explain the fact that I was still alive and well by suggesting the cancer was following an indolent course, which was not something I could remember him mentioning as a possibility during our consultation. The explanation appeared to completely ignore the finding of a very limited and confined amount of cancer during the operation at the City and Royal.

"I told you you'd just get a load of whitewash," I said to Mike after we'd both read the letter.

"Well, it was just a shot in the dark," Mike replied.

"So you're going to drop it now?"

"It's not worth pursuing it further. It won't do any good."

"Well, I'm going to take it up. I think we might have Oswald on the run. It strikes me he was given information about my condition that just wasn't true, and we know who did that, don't we? He just didn't bother to carry out his own investigations, unlike Prof Shaw. He believed what Ellman had told him, and why shouldn't he? Consultants would normally believe and trust each other, wouldn't they? Ellman has been lying about my condition to protect himself. To take it to extremes, he was prepared to condemn me to death to cover up his mistake, whatever it was."

"Now you're going a bit far," Mike butted in.

"I'm not. You think about it. If we hadn't pressed for a referral to the City and Royal, something Oswald seemed reluctant to carry out, that abscess would have burst, and I would probably have died. Ellman is truly evil. If there's any way to get him, we've got to do it."

"But you're suing Foyle now."

"I know, I know, but I still think something might come to light to prove Ellman is the real culprit. Someone will squeal."

"Oh yeah?" Mike looked sceptical. "Well, you do what you want to do, but I don't think it will get you very far."

I wrote back to the Chief Executive stating that my husband and I were very dissatisfied with his reply. I pointed out that without a biopsy, which I was surprised Oswald had not requested, there was insufficient evidence for extensive inoperable cancer. I added that prior to seeing Oswald, Mr Harcourt had told me that from the scan alone, he could not tell whether or not the mass was cancer, only the high CA125 reading suggesting that it might be. I asked how 'can't tell if it's cancer' could become 'incurable cancer' within six days. I also pointed out that Oswald had said he thought I already knew I had incurable cancer. I asked who he thought was meant to have told me this. As I composed the letter it became increasingly obvious to me that Oswald had received information from someone, but that Harcourt had not, or if he had, had chosen to ignore it. As Mike put it, people hadn't been singing from the same hymn sheet. And the writer of the hymn sheet? Ellman, of course. I concluded my letter with a demand for further explanation and an apology for an inaccurate diagnosis.

Back came a reply requesting that I give permission for them to see notes from the City and Royal and Titchmouth hospitals. I did not give permission on the grounds that they were irrelevant for investigating a prognosis given in October 2002 before I had contact with either of these hospitals. I suggested that the fact that I was alive and well nineteen months after the prognosis was sufficient proof of its inaccuracy.

For some weeks nothing happened, so in early June Mike took up the matter again, writing directly to Dr Oswald rather than the Chief Executive, and threatening legal action for the trauma caused unnecessarily to both of us unless a reasonable explanation was forthcoming. The letter was obviously passed by Oswald to the Chief Executive as he once again wrote requesting records from the other hospitals. Mike wrote back saying the request was not justified as our inquiries concerned an incident that happened in October 2002, and nothing more. Basically we wanted to know how Oswald was able to diagnose incurable cancer without a biopsy. Where was the evidence in October 2002 for such a diagnosis and gloomy prognosis? We also wanted to know who was meant to have already have told me of this condition before my consultation with Oswald.

At last, on the 19th of June, nearly three months after Mike's initial inquiry, we received a reply which addressed the issues raised. Oswald claimed that he had not told me the cancer was inoperable, but that surgery would be of limited benefit. He did not suggest a biopsy at that stage because I was being referred to Prof Shaw. That struck me as a very feeble excuse. I still thought he had no right to make assumptions about the seriousness of my cancer without a biopsy. As regards his assumption that I already knew about my condition, he claimed that as I had had this condition for twenty years, I must have known about it. That was complete and utter balderdash. The briefest glance at my records would indicate that for most of that period I was regarded as cured, not even having checks after 1987. Even since 2000 I had received reassuring information, such as only slight borderline changes in material removed. This was miles away from 'extensive incurable cancer'. It was becoming increasingly obvious that someone, and I strongly suspected Ellman, had played up the cancer aspect to cover up other things. However, even if Oswald was now fully aware of what had been going on, he was obviously going to keep it to himself. We were just faced with yet another coating of impenetrable whitewash.

So much for putting pressure on Oswald," I commented to Mike. "We've just gone up yet another dead end, haven't we?"

CHAPTER 23

While we had been pursuing our own little sideline, Bentham had obtained a draft report from Jonathan Muir, the gynaecologist recommended by Prof Shaw. Towards the end of May I received a copy, and as I read it through, it became obvious that Muir was so disgusted by my poor treatment at Casterbridge Hospital that he felt duty-bound to include comments about it in the report although his instructions were to concentrate on the effects of Dr Foyle not referring me to a new consultant. I suppose, quite rightly, he felt it necessary to review the entire picture.

He had done an extremely thorough job and as I slowly read through each section I began to feel that the report might include input from another source. Muir appeared to be making observations and assumptions that could, possibly, be unjustified if drawn only from the material at his disposal. It made me wonder whether he had received some strictly unofficial information from Shaw. After all, the two of them certainly knew each other well, being in the same specialisation – gynaecological oncology. Shaw had recommended Muir to Bentham, and had made the point that it would be inappropriate for him, Shaw, to be involved in the legal action as he was still treating me. Yes, it was quite possible the two of them had had an informal chat about my case.

Soon after I had received the report, Bentham was on the phone about some minor point. Inevitably, we soon got on to Muir's report.

"We're very pleased with it," I commented.

"I'm amazed," Bentham replied. "It's so damning compared with the Jessop report. In all the time I've been working in medical litigation, I've never seen such a divergence of opinion between independent experts."

"Really? Well, I did often wonder what Jessop was up to."

"If we'd had this report from Muir instead of the Jessop report, I think Jeremy Carr would have been more confident in pursuing the case against Casterbridge Hospital and Ellman."

"I suppose it's too late to go back to that."

"Very difficult. For one thing, we're now out of time seeing we're talking about things that happened in 2000. Despite this latest report, I still think you have a better case against Foyle than you have against the hospital."

"What if, in his defence, Foyle tries to move the blame back to the hospital? What would happen then?"

"Er, that's unlikely. We'll cross that bridge if we come to it – big 'if'. Anyway, Jeremy Carr, your counsel, now has the draft report. He may want some minor changes, but I think in the main he'll be pleased with it. It will be interesting to see whether or not Foyle will defend the action. That will be the next development, so I'll be in touch as soon as I hear anything. Meanwhile I'd like your written comments on the Muir report which could help Jeremy Carr in his assessment."

So I was back on my word processor going through the report section by section, making minor corrections and expanding on certain points. As always, it seemed to take forever. As time went on, I was finding that my memory of events was occasionally becoming hazy, and I had to make constant referral to my diary. Although this enabled me to check date accuracy, my entries weren't always detailed enough for me to recall clearly exactly what was said at my numerous consultations with various medics. In fact, Muir's report was so good, my own comments were quite brief. I tried to move right away from my unprovable 'foreign object' theory, which seemed logically to lead to the assumption that it was my own borderline cancerous material which had been left in me after the February 2000 operation, despite Ellman's assurances that he was 99 per cent certain he had removed all such material. If Dr Foyle was aware that potentially cancerous material did indeed remain in me, his negligence in not referring me to a new consultant was very serious indeed. This was the view taken by Muir, and he speculated that had I received prompt referral in 2001, the chance would have been that the cancer would not have developed, and that a permanent colostomy might not have been necessary.

Deep down, I still didn't believe that this was the correct scenario, even though Muir had appeared able to construct an excellent case to prove it with the facts at his disposal. So why couldn't I fully embrace it and forget all about 'foreign objects'? Was I in some kind of denial about my condition without even realising it? I knew that one way cancer patients deal with their disease is to deny its existence, passing it off as something less serious. Doctors recognise this and accept it. But really I couldn't believe I could react in this way, even subconsciously. I liked things straight and honest. I liked to know my enemy and face the danger head on. That was me.

It occurred to me that all along I had been faced with two possibilities - firstly that something had gone wrong after the first operation but had been covered up and put right during the second operation. Further trouble had then started to develop about eighteen months later; secondly that both operations had been unsuccessful and that the medical profession had deliberately conspired to deny me the monitoring and/or treatment I needed. Surely, of the two scenarios, the second was the less likely. The first was the case of a surgeon hiding an unfortunate error - appalling but understandable behaviour. The second was just simply inexplicable, inexcusable, and unbelievable. Take your pick!

Much as I would have liked to have reactivated the case against Ellman, I took on board Bentham's views on the matter. He backed up his remarks on the phone with a long letter about the time limitation problem, and the considerable uncertainty about the outcome of the action and how, if I lost, I would be facing legal bills running into six figures, as I would have to pay the other side's costs as well as my own. Carr's advice, once he had seen the report, was much the same. However, he was optimistic that I would be successful against Foyle, rating my chance of winning at over 66 per cent. His recommendation was that this was the course the case should now take.

Although I suspected I was suing the wrong person, I felt I had to go along with this. Having already spent so much money, I had to go on with the case in an attempt to recoup it, plus a good deal more, I hoped. I also still wanted the truth. Perhaps, in his defence, Foyle would let something slip, something that might land Ellman right back in it. I could always hope. The possibility was there.

The Muir report, although good, had resulted in a period of confusion both for myself and my legal advisors. In fact, Carr's opinion was that the report had some very unexpected aspects. No doubt he too felt I was suing the wrong person, as Carr knew about Ellman's reputation as well as Bentham. I think they would both have liked to have gone for him again. But for me the way forward was clear. I simply couldn't take on the financial risk of suing Ellman and losing. There simply wasn't the firm evidence to prove the wrong-doing which everyone seemed to suspect. A clever lawyer, and Ellman probably knew plenty of those – he needed to – would get him off. My financial outlay had already gone way beyond what I had anticipated. My money wasn't exactly running out, but as there was still some way to go, I did begin to wonder if I was throwing good money after bad. It was time to see whether I could get a conditional fee agreement from Jeffreys and Rowe.

Conditional fee agreement is the proper term for a no-win no-fee arrangement. It is normally only made when a firm considers a client has a very high chance of success in a case. If granted a conditional fee agreement, I would not have to pay any more fees for the duration of the case. I would, however, have to pay the costs of experts' reports and any other incidental expenses. And I would have to pay the other side's costs if I lost, although it is possible to insure against this eventuality. Assuming I did win my case, the fees for my side would be doubled and charged to the losing side. I could immediately see that if a client was on a conditional fee agreement, the opposing side would be forced to recognise the shakiness of their defence, and therefore be anxious to settle quickly to stop the inflated fees from escalating.

When I asked Bentham if I could have a conditional fee agreement, he didn't say yes, but he didn't say no. Instead I got a lot of waffle about the firm's risk assessment officers having to consider the case. Carr's views on the matter would have to be considered, and so on. However, I filled in the appropriate forms, and a few weeks later I got my conditional fee agreement. It seemed that Carr's assessment of winning chances of 66 per cent had been a little pessimistic, and he secretly thought the chance was about 75 per cent. That, it seemed, was good enough for Jeffreys and Rowe to risk not getting any more fees from me. It was a great relief to be free of the constant drain from my savings which I had endured for the past eighteen months. I was not expecting to have to pay for any more expensive reports, so except for some minor court fees for time extensions and the like, I didn't foresee any more major expenses. I decided not to insure against bearing the costs of the defence should I lose because the premium was enormous, and the risk small.

After what had been a confusing period, the way forward was now clear. Jeremy Carr started work on the Particulars of Claim to be served on Dr Foyle. This involved further minor reports from Muir and Read and making sure my most recent medical records were available to them. I think Carr was very much aware that my condition could change for the worse at any time, as medical science could not predict the progress of the cancer. I was having regular monitoring at Titchmouth Hospital. The CA125 blood tests remained within normal limits although there was a slight upward trend. CT scans showed that something slightly suspicious remained in me, although the oncologist could not be sure whether it was a tumour or scar tissue. Between scans it had expanded a little, but only by millimetres. I got the feeling I was a bit of a medical mystery. If it was ovarian cancer, I was told it was a most unusual kind, as most ovarian cancer is aggressive. As far as I was concerned, I felt completely well. The colostomy generally behaved itself, and I just got on with my normal life.

On the 2nd of June 2004 I had another appointment at the City and Royal. Unfortunately I didn't see Prof Shaw. I'd been rather hoping I would as then I'd be able to brag to Goldilocks that I'd been in the presence of the great man and make her jealous. Another doctor on his team checked the most recent scan report from Titchmouth and examined me. He seemed well pleased, and didn't appear to expect any trouble in the near future. Full of the joys of early summer, I made the best of the rest of my day in London testing out the new millennium bridge and photographing the latest weird addition to the city skyline – the Gherkin.

On the strength of the medical view from the City and Royal, Mike and I went ahead and booked a month's holiday in Australia for September. We had intended going in 2003, but that had been out of the question. I was anxious to fit it in as there was always the possibility my health might change for the worse. I had lived and travelled in Australia for six months in 1973 and wanted to revisit some of the places I'd stayed at, and see others I'd never reached such as the Great Barrier Reef. Mike had never been. Throughout our married life exotic long-haul travel had been our principal luxury, but I knew that health insurance was now going to be a problem because cancer and cancer-related symptoms would not be covered as they were a pre-existing condition. Every time I ventured outside the EU countries where reciprocal agreements offered some protection, I was taking quite a risk. I would also stand to lose money if I had to cancel due to cancer-related problems, so would have to book at the last moment and keep advance booking to a minimum, not always easy with complicated long-haul holidays. This was an area where a good financial settlement would give me some peace of mind.

While Bentham and Carr laboured over the Particulars of Claim, I had to prepare a Schedule of Loss which would detail all the losses and expenses my ill-health had caused. I would be able to claim for these in addition to any lump sum awarded by way of compensation for having a permanent colostomy, cancer, and the possibility of cancer recurring. Possible future expenses and losses also had to be calculated which was like staring into a crystal ball and working on the worst possible scenario.

I was sent leaflets with various headings I had to consider. For many people, the principal loss would be earnings caused by sick leave or permanent job loss. However, Mike had retired from his full-time accountancy practice in 2000, soon after my first operation due to his own ill-health. I had retired at the same time. I couldn't therefore claim loss of earnings from that source. But I did have a very small part-time business giving slide shows of my travels to various organisations around the town. I had had to cancel many booked shows during the last few years, but the actual monetary loss was only a few hundred pounds as I only charged £20 a show.

Expenses were slightly more straightforward. Travel was a major heading. I had made numerous trips to various hospitals and with the help of my diary I was able to recall them along with the mode of transport and the cost. Trips to the City and Royal had involved coach and tube fares and the occasional taxi except when I was so ill that I got a free hospital car. Attendance at Titchmouth Hospital involved a seventy-mile round trip by car for which I could claim a set mileage allowance. It soon added up to a good few hundred pounds. As everyone knows, despite the NHS, being ill isn't cheap.

Another major expense had been household and garden help. I normally did all my housework and gardening, Mike being pretty useless in both areas. But after my operations I had needed temporary help both from a domestic cleaner and a gardener – another few hundred pounds.

There was a further heading for miscellaneous expenses, and here Bentham suggested that I should consider such things as necessary new clothing. He seemed to think that a minor change to my anatomy due to the colostomy bag would be an excuse for a complete new wardrobe. However, I hadn't had to buy anything as all my existing gear fitted OK. The only type of clothing unsuitable for a colostomist is tight hipster trousers, and as my trousers were all of the loose-cut elastic-waisted type, they were all comfortable. OK – I would never wear my bikini again, but to be truthful, I would never have worn my bikini again even without a colostomy! I got the feeling that Bentham was basing his assumptions on experience with his wife after her affliction.

The real problem area was future expenses. I put in a notional allowance for future travel for check-ups which would continue for many years. I expected that any future treatment would all be on the NHS, so I couldn't really claim anything under medical expenses. It was impossible to calculate how much household and garden help I would need. I was feeling fine and back to doing everything myself, and I hoped very much that that would continue. However, Bentham urged me to consider the worst possible scenario which would be that I would become totally incapacitated, or even die, in which case Mike would be entitled to the cost of the care I could reasonably be expected to provide for him for his expected lifespan. As he was ten years older than me, the likelihood of me dying first would have been minute in normal circumstances. He would need a part-time housekeeper and gardener. It worked out that this item alone far exceeded all the other costs put together, bringing the total claim to around £30,000. It didn't seem quite right to me. I thought it would be better to only have a right to claim this sort of cost if it actually became necessary, but Bentham said settlements didn't work like that. Despite the fact that I had inflated my claim by as much as my conscience would allow me, he still seemed to think it was on the low side. Anyway, along with the sum expected for compensation, we were now talking about a settlement of at least £70,000. It seemed a lot to me, but possibly wasn't a great deal as medical claims go. Had I been forced to retire from well-paid professional employment, it would have been very much higher.

The Particulars of Claim were eventually served on Dr Foyle in late July. The final document ran to eight pages but the gist of it was that Foyle had been negligent in not acting on the letters he had received from Ellman asking Foyle to arrange for my on-going care. It consisted of a number of points about what he had failed to do, such as discussing the situation with me. In the following section on my personal injury it stated that because of the complete lack of care I had developed further problems resulting in a permanent colostomy being necessary, and the development of cancer needing chemotherapy. It was Muir's opinion that I would have suffered neither of these complications had I received prompt treatment in 2001. Of course, no one could really be certain of this, but in civil law, balance of probability is good enough to win a case. As virtually every medic would agree that the sooner cancer, or potentially cancerous growths, are treated, the better the outcome, I couldn't see that there could be much argument that the two-year delay in my treatment was detrimental.

It was now a question of waiting for Dr Foyle to respond. Would he try to defend his non-action? Did he have any kind of defence? I couldn't think of one. Perhaps he would be advised to immediately admit his shortcomings and negotiate a quick settlement. The thing that intrigued me most of all was would he, in an attempt to defend himself, expose Ellman's role in the affair – a sort of naughty little schoolboy saying "Please miss, it wasn't just me."

CHAPTER 24

Dr Foyle was, of course, covered by one of the big medical insurance companies. Assuming I won my case, there would be no trouble in getting the pay-out. The sort of amount I was claiming was pocket money compared to some settlements they had to meet. His insurers appointed the London solicitors Burnham Brown, and I soon heard from Bentham that a Miss Vera Stone was handling the case. We were quickly informed that they proposed to defend the claim, but Bentham told me that this was normal at this stage of the proceedings. I had a sneaking feeling that he too was expecting a quick settlement. Even so, Bentham had to assume that the case could end up in court, so together we worked on my draft statement which would form the basis of my evidence in court. He also requested a statement from Mike and from another family member or close friend. For the latter I decided to ask my long-standing Scrabble friend, Lena. We'd worked and played together for fifteen years, founding and running the Sandcliffe Scrabble Club. She was a retired teacher and quite extrovert. Anyone who could perform as well as she did in TV quiz shows would not be intimidated in court if she was asked to give evidence. Fortunately she agreed to prepare a statement along the lines suggested by Bentham.

My statement finally ran to fifteen pages. It had to include details of all health problems since 1981 – every consultation, operation and treatment at all of the hospitals I had attended – Casterbridge, Sandcliffe, Titchmouth, and the City and

Royal. Yes, it was complicated. I particularly had to mention my contact over the years with Dr Foyle, seeing the action was against him. Considerable redrafting was necessary here to take into account matters raised in Foyle's defence – more about that later. Then I had to justify the losses and expenses I was claiming, such as household and garden help, travel, and the notional cost of all the hours of care provided by Mike after my 2003 operation.

Mike's statement was much shorter and was mainly to do with confirming my own statement and adding a few points from his own memory of events. He too had to do some redrafting after we had obtained Foyle's defence statement.

Lena's statement was very much shorter, but emphasised the change she had seen in me from an individual of robust health who had worked as her gardener, to a semi-invalid who appeared rather anxious in social situations on account of problems associated with my colostomy. She also mentioned the distress I appeared to suffer due to the confusion surrounding my case.

Throughout August 2004 there was frequent correspondence between Miss Stone and Bentham. It seemed like delaying tactics were being used. There was criticism that some of my medical notes appeared to be missing. Bentham had used a specialist firm to get them ordered into a paginated file, but because they were so voluminous and from four different hospitals, it was difficult to present them in a logical and easily understandable way. The court then had to grant an extension of time for the defence to be prepared. This, in fact, suited me, as I would be away in Australia for the whole of September.

The first inkling of the direction the defence might take came in the middle of August when Miss Stone indicated that they might want to arrange for me to be examined by both a gynaecological oncologist, and a psychiatrist. So were they going to try and prove I was some kind of a nutter? They'd have a job. I felt they were clutching at straws. Perhaps it was just a threat intended to disturb me. They'd think the better of it, no doubt, so I put it right to the back of my mind as I prepared for my month of touring in Australia. They were also insisting on having details of the complementary treatment I had been receiving on an occasional basis from Terry Sutton. I could not see how this could help with the defence case because conventional medics would not understand it. The general view would, no doubt, be similar to Prof Shaw's – that it was unlikely to have had any beneficial effect except possibly as a placebo. Again, I felt they might want to use it to try and prove I was nuts – rejecting conventional treatment in favour of unproved alternatives. I felt I was on pretty safe ground there, as except for a very brief period in spring 2003 when I postponed the operation, I had always stuck to conventional medicine, regarding Terry's treatment as an extra which might have done some good, and certainly didn't do any harm. These days many patients seek additional complementary treatment. Some doctors and hospitals provide certain types on the NHS. It is not considered particularly odd.

I put all my worries in a letter to Bentham. I explained that I thought psychiatry was a very inexact science which could be used to prove anything. I pointed out that if Foyle suspected I was mentally deranged at the time when the relationship with Ellman broke down, he should have done something about it. I had not put much emphasis in my statement on the psychological damage my poor treatment might have caused because there was more than enough physical damage for a good settlement. It was not really necessary to open up a whole new area. But if that was what the defence was going to do, I was going to have to respond. I could envisage top consultant psychiatrists arguing about whether I'd been nuts all along, or whether my appalling medical treatment had had a severe psychological effect. I didn't want to go down that route.

My suspicions about psychiatrists were perhaps a little surprising seeing I actually had one in my family. A second cousin who had become disillusioned with general medicine had moved into psychiatry. I very seldom saw him, but he always struck me as a bit odd. At one time he kept two pythons in his airing cupboard. They were allowed to slither around his flat, coiling up wherever they wanted to. It's all very well to find a cat curled up on your duvet, but a snake? It's normal not to like snakes, not particularly abnormal to be really scared of them, and very odd to keep them as household pets. I rest my case.

Bentham replied in a reassuring tone. He pointed out that even if the defence relied on a psychiatric report to show that I would not have agreed to see a new consultant, this would not excuse Foyle's failure to act on instructions received from Ellman. Bentham was also doubtful that an attempt to show I was relying too heavily on complementary medicine would help the defence. He seemed to think that so long as my statement addressed the issues, and we had a psychiatrist's report to balance the one from the defence, the judge would rule in my favour if the case came to court.

On my return from Australia at the end of September, I found that in my absence Miss Vera Stone had arranged for me to be interviewed by a consultant psychiatrist. I was to see a Dr Pierre De'Ath at his consulting rooms in Titchmouth on the 12th of October. I really hadn't been expecting this because I thought it was just a hollow threat from the other side. Quite unnecessarily, I became a little panicky. I wrote to Bentham pointing out that to produce an effective report for the defence, the psychiatrist was going to have to prove my state of mind in April 2001, three and a half years ago. I didn't think this was possible, and that any decent psychiatrist would point this out. I suspected that information would be twisted and interpreted in a way favourable to the defence. I said that I was going to answer questions very cautiously and that Mike would come with me to take notes. I asked whether it was permissible to tape-record the interview, or even to do it secretly. Bentham wrote back promptly advising that experts did not like their interviews being taped, and if I was discovered recording it secretly, he could refuse to have further dealings with me. That, of course, wouldn't help my case. I could also envisage possible technical problems. Cassette tapes only ran for forty-five minutes per side and I felt sure the interview would last longer than that. The recorder would stop with a loud click, and I would be found out. I'd have to rely entirely on Mike's note-taking ability.

The day of the interview with Dr De'Ath finally arrived. What a name for a doctor! The apostrophe and capital 'A' fooled no one. Why hadn't he changed it? And Pierre! Was he French? I hadn't much time for the French. In general, I found them arrogant and unfriendly. All these thoughts were going through my mind as we sped along the motorway to Titchmouth. We arrived a little late because there was nowhere to park within the vicinity of his consulting room. The limited parking space around the old house was entirely taken up by the posh cars of all the consultants using the building. The needs of patients hadn't been considered. There were no public car parks nearby, and the street parking was all taken. In the end I had to park in the drive, so blocking in all the posh cars. Needless to say, I had to go and move it half way through the interview to let someone out.

A receptionist showed us into his room. My first impression of Dr de'Ath was that he was small in stature and rather weedy-looking with a straggly goatee beard. He conformed entirely with the mental picture I'd built up of him, based, to some extent, on my distant cousin. But at least he was totally English, despite his name. We all sat down and Mike balanced a yellow legal pad on his knee, pen poised. Dr De'Ath had a pad on his desk.

He began by checking details such as my name, age, address,

and present and previous occupations. Before proceeding further I asked him the purpose of the interview. He replied that it was common practice in cases of medical negligence, and in my case it was also to assess my attitude to alternative medicine. Mike started making notes, and we moved on.

"Where were you born?" he asked.

"Kent."

"And what was the occupation of your father?"

"Refrigeration engineer. My mother didn't work – they tended not to in those days."

"Are your parents still alive?"

"No, both dead. My mother died aged 61 and my father at 84."

"Do you have brothers and sisters?"

"One sister four years younger."

"And what does she do?"

"As little as possible – mostly household cleaning." I really couldn't see the relevance of all this personal information, but it wouldn't help me if I wasn't polite and co-operative.

"Is there any history of mental illness in the family?"

"Not that I know of. If there is, they're keeping very quiet about it." I wondered whether I should mention my weird second cousin who was a psychiatrist and kept snakes – I thought the better of it.

He went on to ask about the family atmosphere during my childhood.

"There were the usual squabbles with my sister, and I thought at the time my parents were too strict, but in reality I think they were fairly normal. There were no marital problems – we were a fairly happy family.

"And what about school?"

"I was quite bright. I passed the eleven plus and went to grammar school. I got 'A' levels and went to London University and got an upper second degree in Geography. I taught for a year and then got a Certificate of Education at Cambridge

University." London and Cambridge, I thought. Top-notch. No jumped-up polys for me. That should impress him.

"Were you happy at school?"

"I didn't much like grammar school. We were expected to conform too much. I was a bit of a rebel. But I loved university because there more independent thought was positively encouraged."

I think he understood exactly what I was trying to convey, and was obviously forming the impression that I was a strong-willed person who didn't take kindly to being pushed around.

"And what did you do after you'd got your qualifications?"

"I decided school teaching wasn't for me so moved into further education where I taught Geography and a little English. I taught until 1983, but took two years out to travel in '72 and '73. I went on the hippy trail to Kathmandu, and in case you're wondering, no I wasn't using drugs. I was travelling to see the world. The drug scene didn't interest me, and that was the case with most travellers. Then I went to Australia where I taught for a term to replenish funds. Then I went to New Zealand and back home across the pacific. After coming home I went off again across the Sahara and Congo Basin to East Africa."

"Goodness, that was most unusual for those days," Dr De'Ath commented.

"Not that unusual. Quite a lot of young professionals took a year off to travel and work abroad in the 60s and early 70s." I knew that De'Ath was younger than me and had qualified in 1980 - I'd looked him up. That was the period when Thatcher was at the height of her powers, the work ethic was paramount, and all young people thought about was making loads of money and getting on the property ladder. It was an awful time to be young. Now, once more, the gap year, either before or after university, is back in fashion, perhaps because the current twenty somethings have learnt of their parents' exploits and want a similar experience before settling down.

"I never regretted my travels," I added. "And being a geography teacher, having first-hand knowledge of the less developed world was quite an asset."

"When did you get married?"

"1977. Mike and I met as colleagues at Casterbridge College when I started work there in 1974 after my travels. We went on working there until 1983. Then we both got fed up with education so together built up Mike's small accountancy practice. Basically I was the dog's body, but mainly concentrated on the financial management, like billing the clients. But we've both been retired since March 2000 because of Mike's poor health. He sold out to his partner, but still does the odd job."

I was beginning to enjoy myself. I felt I was coming across as a well-organised highly educated academic with added business skills. I was also adventurous and street-wise. I wasn't someone to be messed with, and I was certainly no shrinking violet.

"Do you have any children?"

"No, and we never wanted any."

Dr De'Ath looked as if he didn't believe me. I'd seen that sceptical look so many times. It's amazing that many people can't accept that some couples, albeit a minority, have no desire to procreate.

"So when I had ovarian cancer in 1981 and the radio-therapy destroyed my fertility, it was no big deal," I added.

"What are your interests these days?"

"Chess and Scrabble and giving audio-visual slide shows about my travels to various local organisations – I'm putting one together on Australia where we've just been."

Dr De'Ath scribbled away on his pad as he went through all the routine questions he probably asked all his patients and referrals.

"Do you drink?"

"Only very occasionally. I've never been a regular drinker."

"And drugs?"

"Unless you count a puff of a joint in Kathmandu, no. As I said, I'm just not interested. I like to keep my wits about me."

"Do you have any criminal convictions?"

I assumed he wouldn't be interested in my 1970 speeding fine, so I said no.

"Have you had any psychological problems in the past?"

"Well, I sometimes get anxious or depressed about things, but don't we all? It's linked to events, and matters usually resolve themselves." I knew very well that anxiety and depression can only be regarded as psychological illnesses if there aren't obvious reasons for them. Anyone who said they never suffered from either would almost certainly be lying, or seriously out of touch with their emotions.

"How would you describe yourself as a person?"

I paused. This wasn't a question, like all the others, where I could reply with the simple facts. I had to be a bit careful.

"I suppose I'd say I'm a bit quiet and introverted, a bit of a thinker. But I'm quite sociable, although I do prefer just a small group of friends rather than a big party. But I'm not afraid of large groups – I stand up in front of audiences when doing my slide shows."

Dr De'Ath turned to Mike. "Would you agree with that?"

"I'd say that's pretty accurate," Mike confirmed.

I hoped I had given the impression that if the case ever got to court, I wouldn't crumble under cross-examination.

At last we got on to my medical history. I had to go through everything, starting right back in 1981 when ovarian cancer was first diagnosed. It was, of course, necessary to voice my suspicions about 'foreign objects' and how Ellman appeared to have covered up his incompetence, otherwise the breakdown of the professional relationship could not be explained. Dr De'Ath seemed rather surprised that the GMC had dismissed my complaint. I explained quite clearly that had anyone made arrangements for me to see a new consultant in April 2001, I would have agreed, although I would have wanted someone in Titchmouth, and I would have wanted them to start from scratch with an MRI or CT scan. At the time, the complete non-action was a clear message to me that I didn't really need further treatment and that therefore my 'foreign object' scenario was correct.

"But perhaps Dr Foyle just forgot to make the referral," Dr De'Ath suggested. "It does happen – pressure of work etc."

"Rubbish! GPs hardly ever have cases of ovarian cancer, perhaps two or three in their entire careers. I'd stick in his mind. And how often do patients have bust-ups with their consultants? That's rare too. I was odd in more ways than one. No, Foyle was in league with Ellman. He knew exactly what had been going on, and was protecting his colleague."

When I'd finally completed the long story, Dr De'Ath remarked, "You've been through hell."

"I agree entirely," I replied. But I was on my guard. By appearing to be sympathetic, he was portraying himself as Mr Nice. I knew their tricks, or thought I did, although in reality I probably knew very little. Interrogators would often make out they were on the side of their victims to try and elicit information from them. I'd have to be a bit careful about what I said and constantly remind myself that Dr De'Ath was acting for the other side.

He asked me how I felt about the whole situation.

"Bitter and frustrated. It's just awful not really knowing what's been going on in your body. It's as if it doesn't belong to me any more. I think the doctors responsible for the negligence should be suitably disciplined. I've clung to the 'foreign object' theory because I still think it's the most feasible, but if I'm wrong on that, it means I was deliberately neglected for no obvious reason. It even seems I was being left to die at a time when a lot could have been done for me. That's a very difficult notion to take on board, which might be why I've clung to the 'foreign object' idea."

Dr De'Ath looked thoughtful but didn't comment.

"Do you sleep well?" he asked.

"Usually, but sometimes I wake up and then the scenarios start swirling round my head and I have a job getting off again. There just don't seem to be any answers, only my theories."

"Are you eating well?"

"Huh! Too well! I've always been overweight. I have to be careful."

"And what about your sex life?"

It's my view that psychiatrists are obsessed with sex, whereas I'm not, far from it. What relevance did it have to the investigation?

"I don't really have one. I've never had much sex drive."

"Did you have other boyfriends before you married?"

What a question to ask in front of Mike!

"Yes." If he was expecting details, he certainly wasn't going to get them.

"Why did you decide to start legal action?"

"Mainly to try and get some answers, but also in the hope of getting disciplinary action taken against the doctors if appropriate. Obviously, I also want to get back the money I've spent on legal fees, but making big sums of money has never been my main intention, as I'm not poor."

"And why are you pursuing Dr Foyle?"

"That was a decision made by my legal team. There's clear evidence against him, whereas there wasn't against Ellman, unfortunately."

"But you appear very well now. What's the point of going on with the action?"

"You seem to forget I have a permanent disability, a colostomy, which can occasionally be very messy and inconvenient. And who knows what the future holds? I could well develop cancer again and die long before my time. Then Mike would have no one to look after him in his old age."

"Right. Thank you. I think that's everything covered."

I was relieved and could hardly wait to get my anorak back on and scarper. The interview had taken one and a half hours. But then Mike spoke:

"You said at the beginning of the interview that you were going to ask Monica about her views on complementary medicine. You haven't done so."

Dr De'Ath looked embarrassed. "Ah, yes, I'd forgotten that. I'll deal with it now. So you had some treatment from a complementary therapist. Could you tell me a bit more about it?"

I tried to explain the best I could about Terry Sutton's combination of homeopathy and acupuncture for both diagnosis and treatment.

"He sort of measures and adjusts various subtle electrical currents in the body," I said rather lamely. "They run through the meridians, you know, those channels used by Chinese acupuncturists. He can sort of balance things to make your own immune system work better. He's been a family friend for many years. He also treated me back in 1981. But I've only ever regarded his treatment as complementary. The only time I relied on his treatment instead of conventional treatment was when I asked for the 2003 operation to be postponed for a few weeks, and that was only with Prof Shaw's approval. But when my kidneys started giving problems I quickly agreed to the op. Perhaps Terry's treatment wasn't effective, but I still think his diagnosis was better than the hospital's in 2002. He said that my body was fighting something but that he didn't think it was cancer, and, indeed, at that time, it was the abscess which was the main problem."

At last we were back in the car heading for the nearest Little Chef for lunch. Bentham was most insistent that I should claim all expenses reasonably justifiable, which was 46 pence a mile for the car, and a meal if I was out for more than a certain time. As my economical little Astra only used about ten pence worth of petrol a mile, I made a nice little profit. Mike and I discussed the interview over our fish and chips.

"De'Ath wasn't really interested in your mental state," Mike said.

I was quite surprised. "Oh? So what was he doing, then? Do you think he had a hidden agenda as it were?"

"He wanted to assess how you'd stand up to cross-questioning in court."

"Really! And what do you think he concluded?"

"That you would be a formidable opponent."

We both laughed.

"But I expect he'll still produce a report to justify his no doubt outrageous fee," I said.

"Of course, but I expect there'll me another short report to Burnham Brown that we'll know nothing about."

"You mean along the lines of 'this woman is totally together, not over-emotional, not likely to crumble, so don't touch her with a barge pole, and settle quickly'. Ha, ha!"

"More or less," Mike confirmed.

"Well, we'll just have to wait and see."

CHAPTER 25

When we got home Mike immediately typed up his scribbled notes while the meeting was still fresh in his memory. I read the draft and added a few points I thought were important, or were needed to clarify matters. I was interested to see that he had added details of the conversation that he'd had with Dr De'Ath while I was moving my car. We had just reached the point in my medical history where we'd been told by Dr Oswald that the cancer was incurable. Mike mentioned how devastated he'd been by the news, but that I had taken it better because I did not believe it as there seemed to be insufficient medical evidence. Whether Dr De'Ath concluded I was a very tough cookie, or had rapidly assumed the ostrich position, I don't know.

I sent a copy of the completed account to Bentham along with my travel claim and covering letter in which I concluded that I couldn't see how a report could be unfavourable to me or particularly favourable to Foyle. I also mentioned Mike's theory that Dr De'Ath had been assessing how I would stand up in court.

Nothing happened until the end of October. Then we received a copy of the defence statement prepared by Foyle and his solicitors. I was surprised that it ran to seven pages. Was there that much to say about the case? What was he dragging up? I sat down at the breakfast table and read it through.

Most of the first part was simply reasonably accurate and uncontentious details of my long-standing relationship with the practice and the treatment I had received since December 1999. But from January 2001, Foyle's memory of events began to diverge considerably from that of my own. He mentioned that at this time, although no actual date was mentioned, he paid a home visit to Mike who was suffering from the after-effects of a gall bladder operation. Foyle claimed that after the consultation he had asked me about the progress of my gynaecological problems. Apparently I had rudely replied that as he had visited to see my husband, I did not want to discuss my own medical problems. I gasped as I read this. It was lies, lies, lies. GP home visits being as rare as hen's teeth, I remembered the occasion clearly. A quick check in my diary showed that it had been made on the 25th of January. I remembered that Foyle, Mike, and I had been upstairs because Mike had to lie flat on the bed while the doctor examined him. When Foyle left he had gone downstairs first and I had followed to see him out. Mike had come down behind me. In the hall Foyle turned to me and said something like, "So you're back". He was referring to the last time he had seen us both at home, about five months earlier. Mike had been suffering from a mental problem brought on by a drug-induced coma when he had had a serious attack of pancreatitis. I got the medics to realise he needed psychiatric help by temporarily leaving him. The help was effective, and I soon returned home. I had told Foyle that everything was OK now. Gynaecological problems weren't mentioned by either of us. Had he enquired about my own health, as he might well have done, I would have said I was well and that I was soon due for another check-up. I would have been quite pleased that he was taking an interest in me even though he had only called to see Mike.

So why had he given such a deliberately untruthful account of the visit? I tried to think what he would have already known about my relationship with Ellman in January 2001. I knew from letters that Ellman had indicated to him that I had been confused about the unsuccessful outcome of the September 2000 operation, and that I had made complaints about the nursing care. But at that stage the breakdown of the relationship had not occurred, and I had no idea that it was going to happen. It had been the events at the check-up appointment in early February which had precipitated that. Foyle's fabricated account suggested that he already knew something he suspected I might know which might have made me act in the distrustful way he claimed I did. He thought I had found out something at that time because he knew full well there was indeed something for me to find out. I had the feeling that Ellman had kept him fully informed all along. Foyle knew all about what had happened in the operating theatre, whatever that was, and he also knew I had accused Ellman of leaving something in me and then surreptitiously removing it.

The next paragraph in the report dealt with the letters received from Ellman which indicated that the professional relationship had broken down and that I had reported Ellman to the GMC. Foyle had dealt with these on the 6th of April 2001, and it was clear that he understood that Ellman wished him to arrange for me to have continuing care elsewhere. But all he did was write in my notes 'see letters from Mr Ellman'. He explained this was done to alert his partners to the existence of these letters should I consult any of them. He then claimed that the letters and my notes remained on his desk for a week or so while he considered how to deal with the problem. Surely all he had to do was lift the phone, dial my number, and ask me to come in to discuss things – about two minutes work. I stopped reading and thought further about things. I knew that one of the letters from Ellman said he would phone Foyle about the situation. I think Foyle was waiting for that call, or trying to contact Ellman himself. The two of them needed to put their heads together to decide if they could refer me to anybody they could trust, or whether it would be safe just to leave me alone. It seemed that they eventually decided on the latter course, but whether that was a reasonably safe course medically, I have no idea. Muir's report would suggest not.

Obviously, what was almost certainly the true explanation for Foyle's non-action did not appear in his statement. I read on, wondering what on earth would come next. Foyle claimed he did much soul-searching, but remembering my reaction to his enquiry in the previous January, or rather the figment of his imagination, he decided to wait for me to contact him. I think he must have been fairly sure this would not happen because both he and Ellman knew that I was completely well at that stage, and intent on following up my complaint to the GMC.

There was even worse to come.

Foyle did not see me again until the 8th of April 2002 when I had a very bad cough and temperature. I was so ill he visited me in bed at home. At the time he diagnosed a lung infection low down in my left lung, although I noticed that in his statement he referred to it as pneumonia. He prescribed some strong antibiotics, and had departed quickly, giving the prescription to Mike who was standing on the landing outside my bedroom door. At the time I had fully expected him to ask if I was having any gynaecological problems, but he didn't, and as I seemed OK in that department I obviously didn't say anything myself. Anyway, I was too ill to talk much. So, that is my recollection of the visit, once again quite clear given that it was an unusual occurrence.

Foyle's account was another flight of imagination. He claimed that he did ask about my gynaecological problems but that again I refused to discuss them because that was not what I had called him out for. He said he respected my wishes. More lies! This was unbelievable! Contrary to what he claimed he did, I had the distinct feeling that Foyle had been anxious to depart as quickly as possible just in case I had indeed raised the embarrassing subject of my gynaecological problems.

The statement went on to outline the subsequent progress of my case after I had consulted Dr Wilson in August 2002. It then reiterated that I had been a difficult patient from the beginning, only reluctantly accepting referral to Ellman in the first place. That definitely wasn't true. Obviously I had been disappointed that my problems appeared serious, but I was grateful for the fast-track referral which Foyle had quite correctly made. Foyle then claimed that had he tried to make new arrangements for me in April 2001, I would not have agreed to them because of the attitude he claimed I showed in January 2001. He thought it best to wait for me to make the first move. What he would have done if I had, I don't know. I imagine he might have tried to persuade me to withdraw my complaint and go back to Ellman. I certainly wouldn't have agreed to that! He suggested I was distrustful of the medical profession, claiming that this was illustrated by my words in a letter to Ellman before the first operation – 'if it ain't broke, don't fix it'. Perhaps Foyle had never heard an old adage quoted to me by none other than Prof Shaw – 'A good surgeon knows how to operate, a better one knows when to operate, but the best knows when not to operate'.

"This is terrible," I said to Mike as I handed him the statement. He frowned, and started to read it while I washed up the breakfast things. Ten minutes later he flung it down on the table.

"Who does he think he is? Hans Christian Andersen?" he said. "I can clearly remember those two visits he mentions. He definitely didn't bring up your gynae problems at either of them. In fact, when you had that chest infection, I was surprised at how quickly he seemed to want to get out. He thrust the prescription in my hand and charged down the stairs."

"Thank goodness you were there during both those visits.

It won't just be my word against his. You did hear what he said, or rather didn't say, on both occasions?"

"Yes, I was coming down the stairs when he spoke to you in the hall, and I was just outside the half-open bedroom door when he was examining you. I could hear him clearly, although I couldn't hear you very well because you had practically no voice."

"What are we going to do? We can't let him get away with this." I was getting quite hot and bothered, thinking people would be inclined to believe a doctor rather than me. But perhaps I was wrong there. Since the Shipman case, people were rather less inclined to place doctors above suspicion.

"Calm down, it's nothing to worry about," Mike said. "We'll both independently write statements about our memories of those two visits. They won't tally exactly which, if anything, will add authenticity. Then we'll send them straight to Bentham. We'll do it now."

"How does Foyle think he can get away with such lies? Would he say these things in court under oath?"

Mike shrugged. "I've got the impression he's a desperate man."

"I've just thought of something," I went on. "If a doctor has an awkward patient who refuses treatment or won't even discuss their condition, a doctor's first thought will be how he will protect himself against possible litigation if the patient becomes ill or even dies. That will come before he thinks how to help the patient see sense. He'd make careful notes at the time in the patient's file. He might try to get a partner or other health professional to act as a witness. He'd make damn sure, at the time, that he could not be blamed. So why hasn't Foyle put something in my notes about me refusing to discuss my problems in April 2002? I've seen the notes. There's nothing there except the diagnosis and what antibiotic he prescribed. I reckon, because there's nothing in my notes, his account won't be believed. He should have thought of that."

"You could well be right. Anyway, let's get on with our statements."

Mike went to his computer and I sat down at my word processor. Firstly I had to calm down and collect my thoughts. Foyle's statement had taken me completely by surprise. Any slight worry I had been harbouring about suing the wrong person had completely vanished. Foyle was a lying, conniving rogue and he deserved everything that I hoped was coming to him. And how naïve I had been in thinking he might spill the beans on Ellman. They were both in this together up to their eyeballs. Admitting to concealing the wrong-doing of another doctor wouldn't help his defence at all. If trying to prove I was nuts didn't work, and I was pretty sure it wouldn't, he would just plead forgetfulness brought on by overwork. Probably nothing much would happen to him.

An hour or so later Mike and I compared our statements. They were almost identical, but differed just a little in minor details, indicating the slight fading of memory which could be expected given the time period involved. I sent them straight off to Bentham with a covering letter. It included the sentences: 'My husband and I are both very distressed to see that the statement contains two blatant lies. We would not have expected this from a professional person'. I went on to point out that probably the best proof for his lies was that there was nothing in my notes about the approaches he claimed he had made.

"Foyle's entire defence is a preposterous allegation," I said to Mike as I sealed the envelope. "And what's more, it's based on blatant lies. You know, I rather hope this case does come to court because I'd like to see Jeremy Carr tearing Foyle apart."

Before Bentham had received this letter I had another one from him informing me that my barrister had now seen Foyle's defence and had described it as 'particularly feeble'. I was delighted, as at one point in my own comments I had described it as 'utterly pathetic'. It seemed that Carr and I were of much the same opinion. I couldn't see how Foyle or his legal advisors could expect to uphold such a defence. Or was I missing something? It wouldn't pay to get too cocksure.

Bentham also took this view, pointing out that Foyle did have what he termed a limited argument and was therefore unlikely to give in. He had sent copies of the defence to my independent experts, Jonathan Muir and Anthony Read, for their comments. Meanwhile Jessop was agitating for his £900 fee for his useless brief report, and threatening to go to the Law Society. Let him, was Bentham's attitude, and I fully agreed.

Dr Read quickly replied that having read the defence, there was nothing he wished to add to his own report. From this I concluded that he didn't think anything that Foyle had stated weakened his own views on the matter. One of the points he raised was that if I had refused referral to a new consultant, this should have been entered into my notes. Muir, following Bentham's request, concentrated on calculating when I could have expected to have had a further operation, had I been seen by a new consultant. He came up with the date of July 2001, i.e. two years earlier than I actually had it. He made the reasonable conclusion having the operation at this time would probably not have resulted in a permanent colostomy, or the development of cancer.

It seemed, therefore, that even though my experts had not been specifically told that Foyle's defence included lies, they both appeared unfazed by his arguments. I had a feeling this was because they simply didn't believe him, but weren't actually going to say so.

The next development was that my case was moved from Casterbridge County Court to Sandcliffe. This was because, Bentham explained, my case was now considered 'substantial' and the larger court at Sandcliffe was more suited to dealing with it.

In the light of Foyle's defence, Jeremy Carr wanted a meeting with both Mike and me to discuss a few changes to our statements. It so happened that he was attending Sandcliffe Court on another matter, so we arranged to meet him there along with Bentham on the 29th of November. I'd never been to Sandcliffe County Court, nor to Casterbridge for that matter. One would expect law courts to be accommodated in a building of imposing architecture, something which stands out as more important among the more mundane civic edifices. Not Sandcliffe County Court. A modern building on the outskirts of town, it has all the gravitas of a unit on an industrial estate. A factory for processing files and red tape I thought as I hunted for a space in the massive car park, except that the workers wear wigs and gowns instead of blue overalls. However, the interior, all done out in light timber and shiny marble-effect floors and walls, did meet with my expectations.

Mike and I, along with Bentham and Carr, all squeezed into a little windowless meeting room. I was slightly amused at how Bentham, a very experienced solicitor, and probably old enough to be Carr's father, seemed to assume the role of humble clerk at these meetings. Carr would turn to him, instructing him to do this, do that, write to so and so, etc, and Bentham would furiously scribble it down on his legal pad. It was evident that the barrister was now very much in charge of the case.

Carr went through my written statement almost line by line, clarifying certain points. He was, no doubt, planning how he would guide me through it if the case came to court. One of his aims seemed to be to sex things up a bit, as fashionable phraseology would put it. Being a naturally reticent person not given to exaggeration, I had not dwelt too much on the less pleasant aspects of a colostomy. Carr seemed to want me to put greater emphasis on my suffering, so I gave him a very graphic and completely truthful account of how the bag had become unstuck while I'd been driving through Sandcliffe in heavy traffic.

"You can imagine the state I was in when I got home," I said.

"Yes," he said, wrinkling his nose slightly. "I'll add this to your statement."

He also went right back to my suspicions about Ellman. Although the case was no longer against him, it was the breakdown in my relationship with him which had precipitated the action against Foyle and it was therefore an important factor. I think Carr wanted to ensure that I had good and logical reasons for my suspicions.

"Can you remember Ellman's reactions when you put your foreign object theory to him?" he asked.

Although the incident had occurred over four years ago, I could remember it clearly.

"He looked sort of shifty," I replied. "He looked down at my notes and shuffled them, as if trying to straighten them." I demonstrated what I meant with the file I happened to have in front of me.

Carr just nodded and looked rather pleased with himself. Like most barristers, he had probably been trained in the interpretation of body language, the apparently innocent things we all do when under stress.

Only the most cursory attention was given to Mike's statement, and none at all to Lena's. As the meeting concluded I felt that Carr was very satisfied with my statement and was almost looking forward to conducting my case in court should it ever get that far. The next big development would be the appearance of De'Ath's psychiatric report, which, although it was now six weeks after the interview, had yet to be produced by the defence. None of us were expecting it to present much of a problem.

CHAPTER 26

We finally received De'Ath's report on the 9th of December, i.e. about two months after the date of the interview. Mike and I both had another long read at the breakfast table, the report running to fifteen pages. I didn't make any comments until Mike had finished reading it. Then I almost exploded.

"So I'm paranoid now!" I stormed. "But what else would you expect from a bloody psychiatrist?"

Mike was somewhat calmer, but obviously concerned.

"It seems like he's scratching around for something, as if he's been instructed to put something against you in it. There seems precious little evidence for his conclusion."

We both looked again at his contentious conclusions. The damning sentences were as follows:

On my belief that something was left in me despite the lack of obvious evidence, he commented, 'It can therefore be considered an overvalued idea or possibly even delusional in nature. Her complaints to the GMC and the Ombudsman regarding Mr Ellman, as well as other complaints about her hospital stay do indicate the possibility of her having developed a querulous reaction which borders on a persecutory delusion. The scope of this, however, appears to be confined to her contact with the medical profession'.

Regarding the possibility of whether I would have been co-operative if Dr Foyle had referred me to a new consultant he surmised, 'I consider it unlikely that Mrs Bland would have attended an appointment with an alternative gynaecologist if

Dr Foyle had made a referral in March/April 2001. I believe this because I consider that Mrs Bland felt alienated from the hospital service and that her paranoia regarding the profession closing ranks would have led her to be suspicious of any other practitioner seeing her at that time'.

"You think what I've been through, what awful treatment I had under Ellman, which has been confirmed in the Muir report," I said. "Wouldn't anyone become suspicious and distrustful of doctors in general? You'd be a bit odd if you didn't. I've reacted in a completely normal way. If you're bitten by a dog, it's normal to be wary of all dogs, even the completely harmless ones."

"Yes, yes, you needn't go on," Mike butted in.

But I did go on. I was furious.

"And this paranoia about the medics closing ranks. Well, they do, don't they? Everyone's been telling me that. Amy, you know, the retired medical secretary, she's always saying, 'They all close ranks, you'll never get anywhere', and she's right. So now they've got the psychiatrist on board. Say anything about 'closed ranks' and you're branded as paranoid."

With a rather dismissive gesture, Mike flipped through the report.

"It's a load of trumped-up rubbish," he declared. "Quite frankly, I don't think you should worry about it too much. It's not strong enough to be particularly harmful to your case. And did you notice how he's got all the dates and events mangled?"

We looked back at the section about my earlier life. According to De'Ath, I had met Mike in 1977, married him in 1983, and then gone travelling round the world with him for two years. I had clearly told De'Ath, confirmed by Mike's notes, that I had travelled in the early 1970s, met Mike in 1974, married in 1977, and set up the practice together in 1983. The inaccuracies did nothing for his overall credibility. I practically doubled up with laughter at the thought of Mike on the hippy trail. He was already settled as a boring little bean counter in Casterbridge when I was seeing the world.

"I wonder what Bentham and Carr will make of it," I said.

"I doubt if they'll be too concerned. Any judge would dismiss it as convenient conclusions with virtually no evidence to back them. It's just a load of nothing really."

I quickly wrote to Bentham pointing out the errors in my chronology and giving my views on the conclusions. I reiterated most firmly that had Foyle suggested a referral to a new consultant, the very action would have made me reconsider my 'foreign object' theory. It had been the total silence from both my GP and the hospital which had strengthened my belief in the theory. Waiting for them to do something had in a way been a test for them. It really seemed that the whole case was going to hinge on my likely reaction if Foyle had raised the issue, so I had to think how I would really have reacted. There was no doubt in my mind that had Foyle called me in 'for a chat' that I would have agreed to see a new consultant at a hospital outside the area. Although my suspicions would have remained, concerns about my health would have been my priority. As my complaint to the GMC was being investigated at that time, I would have been reluctant to be seen as being uncooperative, because if the GMC got to hear of it, I'd have been quickly dismissed as a nutter. Thinking things through, I really could put my hand on my heart and say that of course I would have seen a new consultant. I would be quite prepared to say that in court under oath.

A few days later Bentham phoned me about a few minor issues regarding my statement, and the general progress of the case. We briefly discussed the De'Ath report.

"We may have to consider getting another psychiatric report to balance it," Bentham suggested.

"So, another session in front of some twit which I'll have to pay for."

"I've still to hear what Jeremy Carr thinks about it. He may have other ideas."

Three days later I received a letter from Bentham with some good news – 'Mr Jeremy Carr, your barrister, is very firm in his opinion that Dr De'Ath's report is inadmissible'. There was also a copy of the letter he had sent to Vera Stone, Foyle's solicitor, asking her to confirm that she would not be relying on the De'ath report. If she intended to use it, a formal application would be made to the court for the report to be declared inadmissible. The grounds appeared to be that Dr De'Ath had not found evidence of any psychiatric illness. Presumably, his rather vague references to 'persecutory delusion' and 'paranoia' were considered groundless. And quite right too.

The letter also dealt with another matter raised by Vera Stone. She seemed to think that we would be so alarmed by the De'Ath report that we might wish to reconsider the case. She suggested 'discontinuance', which meant both sides would call an end to proceedings and bear their own costs. Bentham was having none of it, and made it quite clear that I wished to continue with the case. If the other side thought this puffed-up psychiatric report would make any difference, they were sadly mistaken.

Perhaps the defence was also reconsidering their position because a few days later there was another letter from Bentham with a cautiously optimistic tone. Vera Stone had phoned him to ask if we had in mind a ball-park figure for settlement. He hadn't given her one for the simple reason that we ourselves had not yet settled on one. He invited me to give the matter some thought. Everything now seemed quite promising, so I quickly did some rough mental calculations. I knew that what was called my general damages for the pain and suffering caused by having a colostomy would be in the range of £35,000 to £40,000. We had already roughly worked out that my out-of-pocket expenses and expected future expenses would be around £30,000. It therefore seemed I could reasonably expect around £70,000. However, a recent scan had shown that the remnant of the tumour still lurking in my pelvis had increased in size by about one centimetre. The doctors were unable to say whether this was scar tissue or the first signs of further cancer. If the latter, I would need more chemotherapy. There would be more suffering and expense, and perhaps serious incapacity or an untimely death, leaving Mike needing household help. My claim would then increase enormously. With my condition being subject to change and on-going, it was a complicated situation. In fact, I worked out a worst-possible- scenario figure which assumed I would die, and that Mike would then need considerable household help for the rest of his expected life, the length of which had already been calculated. The total figure came to just under £200,000, a large part being for Mike's care – a housewife really is worth her weight in gold! I knew I couldn't expect anything like that, but it was an eye-opener to work it out.

I sent the calculations off to Bentham. It was at this point I finally decided to let him know that I knew his wife had also been a victim of Ellman. I explained that I had seen a newspaper report about the court case, and a further feature about him and his wife winning a cruise confirmed what I had suspected. I suggested that Ellman's concern about Bentham's wife's case may have led to him deciding to cover up whatever mistake he had made with me. I headed the note 'private and not for filing'.

It was now nearly Christmas, so everything went quiet for a while. Despite what might be regarded as setbacks caused by the lies in Foyle's statement, and the exaggerations in the De'Ath report, I was feeling quietly optimistic, a feeling shared, I believed, by my legal team. I didn't think the case would reach court. In one way I felt relieved about that, but in another way I was sorry. If the case was thoroughly examined in front of a judge, I suspected more would come out. Jeremy Carr would give Foyle such a grilling that he might let something slip about what Ellman had been up to. Mike told me a judge has considerable powers, and could ask for what he might consider unsatisfactory or confusing aspects of a case to be investigated further. Perhaps he would smell a rat and ask the GMC to look into matters. The GMC might not have listened to Monica Bland, nobody housewife, but they would listen to a judge. But this was all idle speculation, just something I indulged in while half-watching all the seasonal dross on TV.

2005 began well. My case, being complex, had been retained by one particular judge, District Judge Hinton. Bentham explained that this was so other judges would not have to acquaint themselves with the complicated facts at each stage of the proceedings; just one judge would see the case through. Judge Hinton had already made an important decision. The De'Ath report had been declared inadmissible in response to Bentham's request based on the argument that the case did not concern psychiatric evidence. It seemed that Judge Hinton fully agreed. It was a major step forward for us, as there now appeared to be nothing on which Foyle could build a defence. The judge's reasons for refusing the report was because I was not claiming any psychiatric injury as a result of the alleged negligence, I was not suffering from a psychiatric illness, and whether I would have accepted treatment had it been offered was a matter for the judge to decide. It all seemed quite logical, and very good from my point of view.

I was glad that I had never made an issue of psychiatric injury. My attitude had always been that the negligence had caused enough physical damage for a good settlement without me having to play the psychiatric card. But I could have done. The whole affair had destroyed my trust in the medical profession, and particularly damaging had been the role played by Foyle, both in his negligence and his subsequent lying in his defence statement. If you couldn't trust your family GP of twenty years' standing, who could you trust? As every family who fell victim to Shipman knows, being deceived by your trusted GP leaves a particularly bitter taste in the mouth. Logic told me that I had been unlucky in being involved with a dishonest doctor on a bad day. Most doctors were competent and decent people, but I knew that forever more an element of distrust would tinge my relationship with the medical profession. There had undoubtedly been psychiatric damage.

Bentham had received a lot of other bumf from the court laying out a timetable for the case. It stated when certain documents had to be lodged with the court, and gave the date of the 29th of June for a pre-trial case management conference. Should no out-of-court settlement be reached, a hearing before a circuit judge had been booked for the week beginning the 5th of September, with four days being set aside. Four days! How could it take four days to decide whether or not Foyle had been negligent in not even trying to refer me to a new consultant? I could just imagine all the pernickety arguments, and rather hoped I wouldn't have to sit through them. It also seemed I couldn't expect a settlement in the near future. The lawyers on both sides would spin things out so as to earn nice fat fees. They always did that, reaching settlements on the steps of the court just before the hearing. I rather suspected that as my legal team were on a conditional fee agreement, they'd end up making more from the case than I would. It didn't seem right, but they were highly trained and experienced professionals who were working hard on the case. Of course they could expect high fees.

So, everything was going well. All that was needed from me now was patience, something, I have to admit, I did not possess in abundance. As I frequently commented to medical staff when appointments ran very late, I'm not a very patient patient. (Is that why we're called patients, because we have to be patient?)

My thoughts temporarily turned away from legal matters on to my health. My recent CT scan at Titchmouth had been sent to the City and Royal for review by Prof Shaw. I had an appointment to see him on the 12th of January, and this time I actually saw him, himself. Goldilocks would be jealous! The trouble was, Goldilocks was off on maternity leave and I didn't know when, or if, I would see her again. After some rather uncomfortable probing into my intimate orifices, Prof Shaw declared that he thought the slight swelling shown on the scan was likely to be minor cystic development. Despite the slowly rising CA125, he seemed to think any cancer was totally dormant. He was clearly of the opinion that he would only operate again if it was a matter of life or death. If cancer did reappear, he said further chemotherapy would be the best treatment. Altogether he seemed fairly satisfied with my state of health, which was reassuring. Although nearly eighteen months had passed since the operation, he remembered it well. No doubt my case had remained in his mind because Bentham had been in touch with him asking how much a private operation might cost if I needed one, so that it could be included in my damages as a possible future expense. Certainly Prof Shaw was well aware that I was deep into litigation, and he had always been most cooperative in helping Bentham on various matters. I felt sure he knew more than he was letting on, but on this occasion I think his guard slipped just a little.

"I remember your operation very well," he said. "Such a dreadful mass of fibroids and adhesions." He frowned and shook his head, which somehow conveyed to me that a lot of the problem had been due to bad surgery under Ellman. Or was that just wishful thinking? You can get fibroids and adhesions in other ways. Anyway, it seemed that cancer had only played a minor role and might not have been discovered at all had not all my removed material been examined.

No sooner had I conveyed this fairly good news to Bentham than I received a letter from him with the bad news that the defence had appealed against the judge's decision to declare the De'Ath report inadmissible. It seemed they were really prepared to fight on this point. After all, it was the only defence they had, even though it appeared so flimsy. Bentham explained that there would now have to be a hearing by the judge in which both sides would present their arguments. Carr had been made aware of the situation, and I assumed he would argue my case. I had never suspected that this pathetically weak psychiatric report would cause so much trouble.

The hearing was scheduled for the 8th of February. I was not expected to attend, but I was disappointed to learn that Carr would not be available. Someone would take his place, and all I could do was hope that this person had a good understanding of my case and could present a strong argument supporting my total sanity. Bentham had also learnt that the defence had obtained a letter from Dr De'Ath to add weight to his report. He took a dim view of this, suggesting it was a sneaky way of adding evidence 'through the side door' as he termed it. It seemed the defence would stop at nothing. A copy of this letter was sent to me. In it Dr De'Ath stated that he believed I could be suffering from a degree of paranoia where the medical profession was concerned, that I believed they were closing ranks on me, and that therefore I would not have acted upon advice had it been given to me. It was all mere supposition. De'Ath had completely overlooked the fact that it was a commonly held belief that doctors closed ranks to cover up their mistakes, and that in many cases it was perfectly true. He also supposed that my worries on this score would have a greater weight than worries about my health, assuming I would have been given information to indicate that my health was at risk. The supposition was absolute nonsense. I would have always put my health first, even if it had meant admitting I had been totally wrong in my accusations about 'foreign objects'.

I wrote back to Bentham stressing that in April 2001 I had no reason to be suspicious of Foyle, as I had only found out about the letters he had received from Ellman in about

January 2003. Therefore, had he suggested I saw a new consultant, I would have accepted his advice without question. I also pointed out to Bentham, that even if the De'Ath report was allowed, it could even help me more than the defence. If it could be shown that Foyle believed I was in an irrational state of mind, it was part of his duty of care to me to try and do something about it.

The hearing was listed for noon on the 8th of February. Another barrister had been found to represent me in the absence of Carr, and Bentham informed me that she was not anticipating any difficulty in ensuring the defence's appeal would not succeed. He said he would phone me about the outcome.

Around lunchtime on the 8th I was on tenterhooks. The hearing was expected to last about an hour, so I expected a call between one and two o'clock. The call didn't come until five o'clock. Apparently the hearing had been quite a battle, but we had won. In a follow-up letter Bentham explained that after over one and a half hours of argument, the judge had ruled the De'Ath report inadmissible, but had given permission for a further witness statement which wouldn't contain any expert evidence from De'Ath. I would be able to respond to this with my own statement, and both statements had to be in court by the 8th of April. That all seemed fair enough. Bentham pointed out that the defence could still go to the Court of Appeal in London, but he doubted whether they would. All costs in the matter were to be borne by the defence.

So at long last the De'Ath report was dead and buried.

CHAPTER 27

On the 17th of February Bentham sent me a copy of Foyle's redrafted statement in which he had placed greater emphasis on what he believed my reaction would have been if he had suggested referral to a new consultant. It didn't differ markedly from his first statement, still came across as pathetically weak, and was still packed with lies. I wasn't at all worried about it, although Carr was busy studying it to see how my own statement should be redrafted in response.

Then, on the 3rd of March, out of the blue, there was a major breakthrough. Burnham Brown had faxed a letter to Bentham stating that they were willing to offer a settlement of £50,000, and that this sum had already been paid into court. Bentham phoned me at once.

"Foyle's solicitors are offering you £50,000 in full and final settlement," he explained.

"Wow! £50,000! So at long last it seems they recognise they haven't got a defence."

"It would seem so. No doubt the judge rejecting the psychiatric report had something to do with it."

"The offer seems a fair one to cover what's gone on to date, but doesn't take account of what might happen if the cancer returns."

"I'd agree with that. Things seem very uncertain at the moment. Possibly that's why they've made this offer now, before you know what might be developing."

"I'll have to think about it."

"Of course you will. We don't have to respond immediately. Talk to your husband about it, and let me know what you think after a few days."

"What do you think I should do? I'm quite prepared to take your advice. You're in a better position to know whether I could reasonably expect more."

"Well, I'll be in touch with Jeremy Carr to see what he thinks, but my initial reaction is to do nothing. This is only a first offer. It wouldn't be unreasonable to expect more. It would also be wise to wait and see what develops regarding the cancer. It might be a good idea to get Muir to do a report on your prognosis."

I conveyed the good news to Mike.

"At last there's clear light at the end of the tunnel," he commented.

"But Bentham thinks I should get more, especially if the cancer comes back."

"Perhaps you could accept the £50,000 but have a clause where you could claim more if the cancer returns."

"Can you do that?"

"I think so. Ask Bentham."

"That would be a good idea. I don't want to have money I don't really deserve, but if I die, you will need an awful lot to pay for all the valuable services I provide for free."

"Huh!"

"It would cost a lot to have someone to look after all your needs, wash and iron all your clothes, do the housework, the gardening, drive you here, there, and everywhere – you'd need a full-time housekeeper to keep you to the standard to which you've become accustomed."

"If you say so."

"Anyway, I'll write to Bentham asking if I could take the £50,000 but leave the door open for more if justified."

Bentham replied quickly to my letter, reiterating that £50,000 was a fair offer to cover what had happened to date, and mentioning that Carr was now considering the matter. He had suggested to Carr that it might be appropriate to accept the sum as a preliminary pay-out until the long-term prognosis was clearer. However, this would require a formal court order to keep the case open, because we would not be accepting the payment as a final settlement. He rambled on at some length about how the offer, although no breakdown was shown, covered my general damages for personal suffering and my special damages which were the expenses I'd incurred due to my ill-health. He ended by suggesting no response was made to the offer until we had received Carr's opinion.

A few days later another letter arrived from Bentham. Letters were now passing between us so frequently that whenever Mike saw an envelope with the Jeffreys and Rowe logo on the mat, I'd get the remark, "Oo, another letter from boyfriend!" This one enclosed a copy of a letter from Burnham Brown explaining that Foyle had not put an expert's medical report into court as requested by the judge because they wanted to save money. Bentham was extremely suspicious about this. He felt it was unreasonable to expect us to make a decision on the offer without seeing the medical evidence for the defence. I wondered whether the report had been done, but was so unfavourable to Foyle that it might even help my case and give grounds for a better offer. It all seemed a bit odd and underhand. I think Bentham smelt a rat. Also enclosed was a statement from Dr De'Ath which the judge had said would be allowable instead of the full report. Bentham had rapidly concluded that it would be of little use, and had made Vera Stone aware of his thoughts. The statement was merely a much-shortened version of the medical report, and did not include comments on my mental state. Bentham also pointed out in his reply, of which he sent me a copy, that the judge had ruled that medical evidence from both sides had to be exchanged by the 11th of March. He explained we would not be in a position to consider their offer of settlement until we had seen their medical evidence.

Suddenly that clear light at the end of the tunnel was dimming. Everything seemed to be going wrong. The early, and not unreasonable offer, coupled with the absence of the defence's medical report, suggested they knew something which we didn't. I looked carefully at the judge's instructions as to how the case had to be handled. Certain information had to be supplied to the court for exchange between the sides at specific dates. The notes stated that if either side failed to comply with the directions, the other party could apply for the case to be struck out. I wrote to Bentham asking if we could do this, and what would happen if we did. As my case progressed, I became increasingly aware of the complications of the legal system, and how little I knew about it all.

Bentham replied enclosing a copy of a fax he had sent Vera Stone on the 15th of April pointing out that in not exchanging medical reports, she was in breach of the court order and that he intended to inform the judge about the matter. I left things in his capable hands, but no medical report was forthcoming.

On the 27th of April we had another meeting with Jeremy Carr, this time at Bentham's office. This was principally to discuss our response to the offer of £50,000, known in legal jargon as a Part 36 offer. It was generally felt that if this offer was increased to £60,000, it would be acceptable as a provisional offer to cover general and special damages to date. However, as in the medical report Muir had stated that there was a ten per cent chance that the cancer would return, the case was a suitable one for provisional damages, so leaving the door open for further claims should these become necessary. We discussed at some length how to assess my needs if cancer did recur. It would be an exercise in crystal ball gazing, and therefore it could be unfair to both sides to award damages based on that possibility.

The following day Bentham faxed our rejection of the offer to Vera Stone along with details of the terms of settlement we would find acceptable. He also gave her until the 3rd of May to produce the medical report. Otherwise an application would be made to the court for an 'Unless Order'. Presumably this would mean that the case would be struck out unless the medical report was produced.

If a provisional order was to be obtained, we would have to prove to the judge that there was indeed a fair chance that the cancer would recur. Bentham therefore asked me to get a letter from my consultant oncologist at Titchmouth Hospital explaining the significance of the rising CA125 level along with the expanding tumour shown in the most recent scan. With the departure of Goldilocks on maternity leave, I wasn't sure who was now officially my consultant, so I wrote to the registrar, a Dr Carter, hoping for a prompt reply.

On the 13th of May Bentham received a faxed letter from Vera Stone, who had not responded sooner to our offer of settlement because she had been on leave. The letter stated that they were taking instructions on our offer. It also conceded that Dr Foyle had committed a breach of his duty of care to me in not referring me to a new consultant. However, they would not accept that there was a causative link between this breach and my current condition. They seemed to think that earlier referral would not have meant me having surgery sooner, and with a more successful outcome. They added that 'causation is resisted on the basis of factual evidence'. What factual evidence, I wondered. They still had not produced a medical report, and a further paragraph in the letter made it clear that they were not going to as it was deemed inappropriate. Bentham, in his covering letter, commented that he found this extraordinary, as the only report they were relying on was the statement from Dr De'Ath which contained nothing of any significance.

Along with Bentham, and, no doubt, Carr as well, I found it all very puzzling. Just about every medic in the world would agree that if cancer is operated on as soon as possible, both the surgical consequences and long-term outcome are more satisfactory. Because of Foyle's lack of action, I had suffered a delay of over two years, and they were denying a causative link. It was totally unbelievable.

With all these thought swirling round my head, I went right back to my original, and still firmly-held belief – the foreign object theory. Foyle knew all about it, of that I was sure. He was therefore right in suggesting, as presumably he had done to his legal team, that I would not have had surgery sooner if he had referred me. It was my belief that there was nothing wrong with me in April 2001. Foyle was probably almost certain of this, because Ellman would have told him so. If cancer was developing, my own feeling was that had I been under another consultant, it would not have been picked up for another year to eighteen months. I might have had an operation rather sooner than I did, but quite possibly the outcome might not have been any better. Foyle knew all this, but unless he was prepared to spill the beans, so revealing both Ellman's incompetence and dishonest cover-up, there was no way he could defend himself on the issue of the causative link.

I wondered to what extent Foyle had been open and honest with his advisors. He might have wanted to reveal all if he was the sort of person who believed honesty was the best policy. But if he was that sort, he would never have gone along with the conspiracy in the first place. No doubt he now had little control over the case. His big medical insurers would be calling the shots, and they would by now have accepted that they were liable, and would be looking for the fastest and cheapest way to settle. If Foyle had even suggested telling the truth, their attitude would have been 'don't even think of going there'. An almighty can of worms would have been opened, and many eminent heads would have rolled. I just had to accept that my partly fabricated medical history was so firmly in place that nothing was going to budge it.

Bentham quickly replied to Vera Stone asking her to cover

the costs he had incurred in obtaining an 'Unless Order' from the court for the exchange of medical reports. He pointed out that he could have been informed far earlier that there would not be one. He also warned her that if there was a trial De'Ath's statement would be objected to on the grounds that it was irrelevant.

I wrote to Bentham expressing my views on the various strange developments. I asked him why they had already made an offer of £50,000 when they were not admitting to a causative link. It seemed rather a lot for a breach of duty of care without serious consequences. In fact, it seemed rather like hush money – Here's fifty grand. Now shut up and go away. I expressed doubts about the morality of accepting any payment without an admission of liability from the other side. I did not say so at the time, but I was certainly not prepared to sign anything like a gagging clause.

Meanwhile, at Sandcliffe Court, Judge Hinton had acted upon Bentham's application for an 'Unless Order'. It appeared that Vera Stone had also failed to inform the court that there would be no medical report. She wasn't exactly endearing herself to the judge, I thought with some satisfaction. Bentham wrote to the court with a full explanation of what had been going on. It seemed to me that everything was getting very confused and that attitudes were now hardening on both sides.

My brain seemed to be in permanent overdrive, always juggling this or that scenario. I'd try to relax by watching TV, but what did I get – a news item about a doctor who had misdiagnosed breast cancer and had tried to cover it up by substituting a diseased tissue slide from another patient for his patient's healthy tissue. It seemed these doctors would stop at nothing, and it brought to the fore an aspect of my own case which had been niggling me for some time, and was connected with my tissue samples.

When Prof Shaw had asked for a re-analysis of my tissue samples to date in-house at the City and Royal, Casterbridge

Hospital had sent them by second-class post, which didn't seem right for important medical samples. Had they hoped they would be lost or damaged? Analysis showed that the diseased cells from the 1981 tissue samples were exactly the same in appearance as those in the February 2000 samples. How likely was that, I wondered? There had been a period of eighteen and a half years in which changes could have been expected to have taken place. There had been a dose of radiotherapy in 1981. Did that cause diseased cells to revert to normal, or did it simply freeze a cell at the level of change already reached? It was a highly technical question, and I had no idea of the answer. Why had the doctor I had seen in January 2000 expressed doubt about whether the 1981 slides still existed? As it seemed they were still available, why had they not been re-analysed before the February 2000 operation? Prof Shaw seemed to think that was important, so why hadn't Ellman? The thought going through my mind was that the 1981 slides were, in fact, made from tissue removed in February 2000. Ellman might have got this done to give the impression that I had an on-going but virtually dormant cancerous condition, whereas I had always thought of it as two separate episodes, the second of which was caught before it got going. But the on-going condition was all part of the false medical history which, it appeared, had been created for me. It explained why Dr Oswald had declared that he thought I knew I had incurable cancer. It also seemed why Foyle was claiming that there was no causative link between his breach of duty and my condition. He would say I was already a hopeless case, and therefore earlier referral to a new consultant would not have made any difference. So perhaps he did have a defence without spilling the beans. But why didn't he obtain a medical report to back it up?

I wrote to Bentham about my concerns. I wondered if it was possible to detect the vintage of tissue slides. Back in 1981 they might have been prepared rather differently from those of today, but only an older pathologist might be aware of any subtle changes. I urged him to consider how a false history of on-going cancer could affect the outcome of the case against Foyle.

Bentham replied with the firm view that, at least for the time being, I should stay right away from any aspect which appeared to suggest conspiracy because it raised the issue of paranoia, something we intended to keep well away from! He pointed out that conspiracy would be a criminal offence, and that therefore there was no time limit on pursuing it. It would be a matter to consider once the civil action was concluded. However, he did appear to take on board that Foyle might use on-going cancer in his defence, and had therefore sent a copy of my letter to Jeremy Carr.

The possibility of a false medical history caused me a great deal of anxiety, as it could have an adverse effect on my future care. I had felt all along that the cancer aspect had been overplayed, and I did have some evidence to support this view. Terry Sutton had never diagnosed cancer with his sensitive equipment, despite having considerable experience of making such diagnoses. He would sometimes pick up cancer in a patient before conventional medical testing showed anything wrong. I was the only patient who had come to him with a cancer diagnosis where he could not find obvious evidence. The closest he had come was that I showed a tendency to be vulnerable to cancer, a weakness reflected in the fact that I had had it in 1981. Then there was the fact that Prof Shaw was prepared to say at one point that he doubted whether I had cancer. It was only after the best part of a fortnight's analysis of my tissues in the pathology lab that any cancer was found, and it would not have been discovered had the material not been analysed. During the operation cancer wasn't obvious to the naked eye of an experienced cancer surgeon – material had only been classed as 'a bit suspicious'. If it was assumed that all my problems were caused by cancer, I could have the wrong treatment, and the possibility of other problems could be overlooked. But what on earth could I do about it?

The next development in the case was that the defence rejected Bentham's suggestion of a provisional settlement of around £60,000. However, they raised their full and final offer to £75,000 and had already paid the extra money into court. For some reason they seemed to be on the run. Was there something getting too hot for them to handle? With all my suspicions about conspiracy and great big cans of worms to be opened, I began to wonder whether they might pay out whatever I asked for. But that would be tantamount to blackmail, and I just wasn't interested. I still wanted truth and justice rather than large sums of money. All the same, I knew there would come a point when I would be advised to settle, but until we had a better understanding of the likelihood of cancer recurring, we could not agree to a final settlement.

Bentham was most anxious for more information from Titchmouth Hospital about my rising CA125 level and growing tumour. A locum consultant, a Sri Lankan with a name as long as your arm, was now dealing with my case. He provided a letter showing that the CA125 had risen from 19 to 116 in nine months. As so many things can cause a rising CA125, it was not, by itself, clear evidence of recurring cancer. Fortunately I had another CT scan scheduled for the 27th of May, and this was expected to make the situation clearer.

After the scan Mike and I went off on a Norwegian cruise. It was a welcome break, but it is impossible to get away from it all when the 'all' is your own body. If I felt the slightest bit off-colour, or unusually tired, as everyone does on occasions, I always worried that it was the cancer returning. My health, and my legal case, were always on my mind.

CHAPTER 28

While I was on holiday the defence requested that the next major development in my case, the case management conference before Judge Hinton on the 29th of June, be postponed for four weeks. Their grounds were that both sides needed to know the status of my cancer to make any progress. They had a point, but Bentham knew I would have the result of the latest scan on the 17th of June, so rejected the request.

On the 17th of June I went to Titchmouth Hospital and saw the Sri Lankan locum. He had such a thick accent that I had great difficulty in understanding him. The news was very bad. My CA125 had risen to 156, and the scan showed a steady increase in the size of the tumour. The conclusion was that the cancer had returned, and that I would need more chemotherapy. Another problem was that the tumour was putting pressure on the ureters which had caused a slight swelling of my kidneys and poor renal function. I would need stents again, as I had in the summer of 2003. It appeared this matter was more pressing than chemotherapy, as I would not cope well with the latter if my renal function was poor.

I briefly explained my legal position, and asked for a letter outlining my current problems which I could give to my solicitor. The locum agreed to provide one as soon as possible. I could now anticipate very substantial damages, almost certainly of at least £100,000. It was time to make use of the money. Before agreeing to any further chemotherapy, I wanted a private second opinion. I had a vague feeling that the locum had put two and two together and had come up with five. He wasn't familiar with my case in the way Goldilocks had been. I'd always had the feeling that she knew rather more about me from Prof Shaw than was evident from their correspondence. How thoroughly had this temporary stand-in studied my notes? Probably not at all. He was just drawing conclusions from the latest information available to him. It would be worth paying a top expert to spend a little more time considering the matter.

I was recommended to consult Professor Malcolm Greenwood at a major cancer hospital in London. Nobody seemed to mind me wanting a private second opinion. In fact, they seemed to welcome it. I think the specialist nurse who helped me recognised that being under the care of a locum consultant wasn't ideal. Once I was back home I phoned Prof Greenwood's secretary and got an appointment for the 4th of July. It was explained to me that the fee would amount to around £250, and that I could pay by credit card. The amount was pretty much what I expected, and I felt it would be money well spent, and money which I could easily afford.

I did, of course, immediately inform Bentham of the latest development as it would have a major effect on the matters to be discussed at the case management conference, now only twelve days away. The reoccurrence of cancer, which had always been regarded as a slight possibility, was now reality. In a way, it clarified matters, but also raised a raft of new imponderables. What treatment would I need? Would the NHS deliver the goods, or would I have to pay if I wanted the best available treatment? What was my life expectancy now, and what help and support would I need during the next few years? What was Mike's life expectancy? Would he now outlive me and have to pay for household help that I would have provided? They were all unanswerable questions, but they had to be faced, and answers arrived at, principally in monetary terms so that damages could be calculated.

Further medical reports would be required. Bentham contacted Jonathan Muir and, amazingly, managed to arrange a meeting with him for the evening of the 22nd of June. He did a rapid phone round and by good fortune was able to arrange for Carr, me and Mike, and himself to meet at Muir's house in Titchmouth at six. Brief reports could then be prepared in time for the case management conference.

The 22nd was a very hot day. We all drove separately to Titchmouth and were all delayed by rush-hour traffic, so arriving hot, bothered, and late. Muir was quite understanding and had laid on tea, or iced water, and chocolate biscuits. We sat down round his dining room table with bundles of notes and files in front of us. As usual, Carr was very much in charge and Bentham took notes. Muir had been forwarded the latest information from Titchmouth Hospital (he worked elsewhere) and had had time to study it.

"This is an unfortunate but very important development," Carr stated. "It will obviously have a considerable effect on the case and the amount of damages."

"I understand that," Muir replied. "I'm sorry to say it does seem virtually certain that the ovarian cancer has recurred."

"And the implications of that?" Carr prompted.

"Mrs Bland will need further unpleasant chemotherapy, possibly a number of courses. However, the slight good news is that there is no evidence of cancer anywhere else in her body."

I looked at him. He seemed a little surprised that the cancer was still confined to a small area of my pelvis when, presumably, I had had it for so long, certainly since 2000, and perhaps even since 1981. Ovarian cancer was usually aggressive. If you weren't cured, you were usually dead well within five years. He went on.

"The rising CA125 by itself isn't reliable evidence, but the latest CT scan report does strongly suggest cancer has returned."

"Would further surgery be necessary?" Carr asked.

"Unlikely, as it wouldn't do much good. If cancer invades the bladder, however, Mrs Bland would need surgery and another bag."

I didn't want to even think about that.

"I'm sorry to have to ask this in your presence, Mrs Bland," Carr said, "but what about overall life expectancy?"

Muir looked vague. "Very difficult to say. Treatments are improving all the time, and if Mrs Bland responds well, perhaps ten years."

I guessed he was being deliberately optimistic so as not to upset me, but he could well be correct in his assessment. Prof Shaw had even suggested something else might carry me off before the cancer did.

I decided it was time to ask a question.

"If I'd been referred to a new consultant in April 2001, would the cancer have been discovered sooner, and treated more effectively?"

"Quite possibly," Muir replied. "The chance of recurrence would have been considerably smaller."

That is what I wanted to hear. I think it had been the question Carr had been about to ask.

"If the probability that the outcome would have been better is greater than fifty per cent, then your case will succeed," he explained. "In civil actions you don't have to prove certainty – it goes on the balance of probability."

Muir seemed quite familiar with all this. "I'd say the balance of probability is very much in Mrs Bland's favour," he stated.

From the point of view of my case, the meeting had gone well. So confident was Bentham that my case would now be quickly concluded, he decided it would be in order to ask the defence for an interim payment of £1750 to cover the cost of my consultation with Prof Greenwood, and the £1500 deposit I would have to pay if I decided to have private treatment from him. The matter would be raised at the case management conference.

This conference, before District Judge Hinton, was to take place on the afternoon of the 29th of June and was the next important date in my diary. I didn't have to attend, but Bentham didn't think it would harm my case if I did, and I was curious to see how the meeting would be conducted. I'd also have a chance to assess the legal opposition. No doubt Vera Stone would be there representing Foyle's interests, and also whatever barrister they had appointed. I doubted whether Foyle himself would be present.

Mike and I met up with Bentham and Carr at Sandcliffe Court at the appointed hour on the 29th and we all trouped into the judge's chambers. It wasn't a formal court, so no one was in wigs and gowns. All the same, Judge Hinton still sat at a bench higher than the rest of us as we sat round a table in front of him – Bentham and Carr to his right, Foyle's representatives to his left, and Mike and I opposite him. I had already developed a mental picture of the judge and Vera Stone. The former would be a grey-haired old fuddy-duddy who would shuffle and mumble his way through the proceedings, and Vera Stone would be an old battle-axe with a stiff perm and even stiffer business suit – a sort of Margaret Thatcher look-alike. I couldn't have been more wrong. Judge Hinton appeared quite young – well, anyone under fifty seems young when you're pushing sixty. He had brown hair with Hugh Grant-style floppiness, and he was pin-sharp, rattling through the business and keeping both sides on their toes. Vera Stone was very young and anorexically thin. She was accompanied by a skinny young man who I assumed was the barrister's junior. They were wearing almost identical black suits and I immediately christened them the stick insects.

Soon a lot of legal jargon was flying back and forth, and I found it impossible to keep up. Certain things had to be done by certain dates, with a timetable running up to the trial scheduled for the 5th of September. Judge Hinton seemed anxious that we should try to reach a settlement without a trial, and wanted to know whether an offer had been made. Carr explained that an offer of £75,000 had been rejected because my prognosis was so unclear. The judge felt that the defence was justified in requiring an opinion from a specialist on the matter before any final settlement could be agreed. Obviously, as a judge, he had to be fair. However, I did get the impression that he had become a little impatient with the defence, and Foyle's representative did look a bit rattled. Glancing across at me, the judge said in no uncertain terms that he thought I had a strong case. Bentham and Carr sat looking quietly confident. The only area where the defence won was in defeating my side's request for an interim payment to cover my consultation with Professor Greenwood.

The meeting lasted about an hour. Before going our separate ways we had a quick chat with Bentham and Carr where it was decided that we must obtain an expert's opinion on my prognosis as soon as possible. The other side would be doing the same. Bentham decided to approach both Muir and Professor Greenwood. The principal evidence would be my most recent CT scan. Through the wonders of modern technology, this could be put on to a CD and quickly sent to wherever it was needed. Bentham worked fast, but quickly drew a blank. Muir didn't regard himself as an expert in the interpretation of CT scans, and Greenwood would not become involved, no doubt because I was about to consult him as a patient.

Bentham therefore had to scour the country for a top gynaecological oncologist who had no connection with me, who was willing to take on legal work (many won't) and who hadn't already been retained by the defence. It was a tall order, but he finally located a Dr Jill Leyton and sent her all the necessary information.

The next important date in my exciting but increasingly

traumatic life was my consultation with Prof Greenwood on the 4th of July in the private wing of a West London hospital. I told myself it was very fortunate that I felt perfectly well despite having a life-threatening illness. If it wasn't for all the tests and scans, I wouldn't have had a clue that there was anything wrong with me. As usual, I took the coach to London, this time getting off at Hammersmith and taking the tube. As I found my way to the private entrance of the hospital, I wondered how things would differ from the NHS. I had never had any private treatment before, excepting my compliementary care from Terry Sutton.

The waiting area was very comfortable. There were soft armchairs, free coffee, and the day's broadsheets. It was a far cry from the plastic chairs, thinly upholstered benches, and dog-eared ancient magazines of the average NHS waiting room, which was fortunate seeing I was kept waiting forty-five minutes beyond my appointment time. That was worse than the NHS where waits usually averaged out at half an hour. I had plenty of time to observe my fellow patients, none of whom appeared to be British. There were a number of figures completely covered in black cloaks and veils. I assumed they were women, but it was impossible to tell when all you could see were two frightened-looking eyes. For all I knew, they could be the wives of Osama Bin Laden. I had last encountered such women on my hippy travels in Afghanistan, but it didn't seem right seeing them in London.

At last I was called. First I saw a drop-dead gorgeous junior doctor who took my history and examined me. Then I met Professor Greenwood, who was grey-haired and slightly cuddly-looking.

"I spent the week-end going through your notes," he said. I guessed that was an exaggeration. He's probably spent half an hour at most jotting down the main points. "So you first had ovarian cancer in 1981," he went on.

"Yes, that's right, and I had a course of radiotherapy."

"Then you had more problems in 2000, when you had the left ovary removed and a hysterectomy, then a second unsuccessful operation."

"But I think something was done during that op because I'd had bowel problems which cleared up afterwards."

Prof Greenwood made no comment. "Then in July 2003 Professor Shaw removed your rectum."

"Yes. I have a permanent colostomy. A little cancer was found so I had six doses of carboplatin."

"Your notes seem incomplete. What treatment were you having between 1981 and 2000?"

Suddenly I felt I was wasting my money. If Greenwood had indeed gone through my notes he would have realised I had been cured in 1981. But somehow he had been influenced by the more recent spin about my cancer being on-going.

"I didn't have any further treatment after the radiotherapy. I had check-ups until 1987 when I was told I was cured."

Greenwood looked at me as if he didn't believe me. Why on earth did he even think I might be lying?

"So you would like me to recommend your future treatment?"

"Yes please. I'm expecting quite a sizeable settlement from legal action against my GP, so I'll be able to afford private treatment, as I want to have what you would consider the best."

"I'm not willing to treat you privately, but I would treat you under the NHS if you wish. However, Titchmouth is an excellent cancer centre and you wouldn't get better treatment anywhere else. You'd do well to remain there."

"I see. So what treatment would you recommend?"

"A combination of carboplatin and taxol. You would need a course every eighteen months or so. You could have up to three courses, and then we could probably use other more experimental drugs. In other words we can keep things steady for some years."

"And I suppose new treatments are coming along all the time," I said with an optimism I didn't really feel.

"Oh yes, the outlook is slowly improving," Prof Greenwood confirmed. "I'll write to your consultant in Titchmouth and recommend that you have carboplatin and taxol. I think it would be best if you continue your treatment there."

And that was that. I'd had my £250 worth, for what it was worth. I didn't feel it had been money well spent. I had expected a more thorough examination of both my notes and myself. It had really been no more than a rubber-stamping exercise. No doubt Titchmouth Hospital would have recommended the same treatment.

I made my way back to Hammersmith and ate my packed lunch sitting on the dried-up grass in front of the church while I waited for the Casterbridge coach. It made sense to have further treatment under the NHS at Titchmouth, I thought. A private course of chemotherapy could cost £20,000. If the NHS could deliver it, it would make sense to take it, even if I did win £100,000 or more in damages. I'd keep that to pay for treatment if the NHS let me down. However, I did wonder why Greenwood had refused to treat me privately. It seemed a bit odd. I didn't dwell on that matter too long because something else was occupying my thoughts – taxol was the drug that made your hair fall out.

Directly I was home I wrote to Bentham about all the latest developments, and we also discussed matters on the phone. He seemed to think I was fully entitled to expect my damages to cover the costs of private treatment whether I had it or not. We already had in mind the figure of £100,000 as a suitable settlement, but this was now raised to £150,000 to £200,000, although it would have to be backed up by a report on my prognosis from Dr Leyton, who would have to be in general agreement with a similar medical report from the defence. I felt at long last we were on the home straight, and that from a legal and financial point of view things had turned out very much in my favour. However, that was only a thin coating of sugar on a very bitter pill.

During our conversation it came to light that Bentham had had some discussion on the phone with Prof Greenwood. It had been principally to establish the private costs of chemotherapy, but quite out of the blue Greenwood had asked why it was thought I would win my case. It seemed he thought the long-term outcome would have been the same whether or not Foyle had referred me to a new consultant. In other words, he did not think there was a causative link. So why did his opinion differ so markedly from that of Muir? Why did two experts with the same information available to them reach different conclusions? Why had Greenwood referred to 'missing records'? I began to think he had received inaccurate information elsewhere which he had believed, but which had not been backed up by my notes. In that case, could I rely on his recommendation for more chemotherapy?

Later on in July I had to go to Titchmouth Hospital to have a stent fitted into my left ureter. This would relieve the partial blockage caused by the mass, and improve the kidney function so that I could cope with a course of chemotherapy. When I had previously had stents put in at Sandcliffe Hospital in 2003, it had been done under general anaesthetic from the bladder end. This time it was done under local anaesthetic and light sedation via the kidney end. Neither measure appeared to work properly. I was wide awake and felt everything. It was like having a long nail banged into me. I complained bitterly about the pain to anyone who would listen, but was met with general disbelief. The procedure wasn't meant to be anything more than a little uncomfortable. I think they thought I was a right little cry-baby, but, in fact, I was anything but. Didn't I have my teeth drilled without injections? My dentist said I had a very high pain threshold. It all made me wonder whether the procedure had been done properly.

While the stent settled down I had a nephrotomy tube in my kidney so that the urine drained directly into a bag. This was removed after a few days, and I was allowed home. Further tests would be needed to see whether the right ureter would also need a stent. Therefore in early August I had a test on my urine flow and it was decided that another stent was needed.

On the 8th of August I again returned to Titchmouth Hospital. This time they put me in the cancer ward. I felt perfectly well, but found myself surrounded by very ill-looking baldies who picked at their food, and were probably on their last legs. Would I be like that in a year or two? Somehow I instinctively felt I was in the wrong place. Was I just in denial, a common coping mechanism among cancer sufferers, or was there more to it? Just how accurate was the diagnosis? Anyway, I tried to make the best of it – at least the bedside TV was free. To get away from my fellow patients I would go and sit in my car in the car park and listen to the stereo. I'd found that I could park for £10 a week which was considerably less than the cost of train fares and taxis.

The next day I discovered that I had been assigned to a new consultant, a Dr Nigel Merton. He came to see me and told me that once the stents were in place and working properly, they would begin chemotherapy.

"We'll give you another course of carboplatin," he said.

"But Prof Greenwood said it should be combined with taxol," I replied.

"I think you'll do just as well on carboplatin alone," he explained.

I wasn't going to argue because if I didn't have the taxol, my hair wouldn't fall out. But it did strike me as odd that Dr Merton was overruling the advice of one of the top oncologists in the country. Did he know something that Prof Greenwood didn't? It confirmed once more that my private consultation had been a waste of money.

While in hospital I would phone Mike every evening on

my mobile. I usually went into a corridor or the day room where I was told it was permissible to use one. I well remember the conversation we had on the 11th of August, as it used up most of the credit on my pay-as-you-go phone. Firstly we discussed a letter from Bentham, which I always allowed Mike to open in my absence. Bentham had received a copy of the report from a Professor Heather Terry, the expert for the defence. He was furious because instead of commenting on my life expectancy and the type of treatment I would need, as she had been asked to do, she had questioned Muir's report on causation. This was an attempt to introduce a defence through the back door, Bentham claimed, and he was sending a copy to Jeremy Carr for his comments. Not having seen the report, I couldn't comment, but it was concerning that there appeared to be a fundamental disagreement among top experts.

The next matter was far more intriguing.

"I saw Wilson this afternoon," Mike said.

Dr Wilson, Foyle's partner, was doing an excellent job in keeping Mike's diabetes stable, which was why he had stayed with the practice. "Just as I was leaving, he asked me what I thought about your case. I said I didn't want to comment. But then Wilson said you were pursuing the wrong person, so I said 'so who should she be pursuing?' and Wilson said something like 'I needn't say – we both know'."

"Ellman, of course."

"But it's far too late to do anything about it. We're on the point of settlement, it seems."

"This is as good as it's going to get. Haven't I always said Foyle knew exactly what had been going on, and that was the real reason he didn't refer me to a new consultant."

"But there's nothing you can do about it."

"Oh no? If this case comes to court, perhaps under oath Foyle will spill the beans. Then the flood gates will open. Everyone will be in it up to their necks – Ellman, Foyle,

Wilson, the GMC, the NHS complaints body, the Ombudsman, the police, Prof Greenwood, Dr Merton, and perhaps even Prof Shaw."

"Dream on. You're not going to get your day in court. In the circumstances they'll be more than anxious to settle out of court."

"I reckon I could get whatever I ask for. It's hush money."

"Maybe."

"But I'm not a blackmailer. I want truth and justice."

"You're not going to get it. Take the money and run."

"But I'm not signing any confidentiality agreement or the like."

"You won't have to. That's never been mentioned, has it?"

We exchanged a few more comments, and after the call had ended I remained sitting on the hideous purple sofa in the day room, everything churning round in my mind. I felt vindicated. Ellman was the principal culprit. What a horrendous mess, what a tangled web. But why had Wilson spoken out? OK, he hadn't gone as far as uttering a name, but he didn't have to. Wilson and Foyle had been partners for many years, and I had always regarded Wilson as someone who was exceptionally moral, and a doctor who would always play it safe, never cutting corners. He was also extremely sympathetic. He knew what had been going on. He knew that to a large extent that Foyle was the scapegoat. He'd watched his partner suffer. Perhaps his action was just a last-ditch attempt to put things right, something to salve his conscience.

CHAPTER 29

With stents fitted in my ureters, I returned home from Titchmouth Hospital. I would attend as a day patient in September to start a course of chemotherapy. Meanwhile I had to concentrate on legal matters as things were now at a critical point. There was every indication that the defence was prepared to settle, and now that the facts were clearer, we were in a position to finalise our claim.

Altogether, both sides now had in their possession no fewer than four reports from eminent gynaecological oncologists. Firstly there was Jonathan Muir's. This dealt largely with the strong likelihood that my cancer would not have developed had Foyle referred me to a new consultant who would then have advised further treatment without delay. He was quite clear that on the balance of probability, there was indeed a causative link between Foyle's breach of duty and my present medical condition. Being principally a surgeon, he had declined to comment on my likely future treatment and prognosis, suggesting this was more the area for an oncologist.

Dr Jill Leyton's report was extremely comprehensive. She included copies of articles from the medical press about the treatment and prognosis for borderline ovarian cancer. It was a problem that my type of cancer made up only about ten per cent of ovarian cancers. On that basis there might only be six hundred or so cases a year in the UK – not and awful lot on which to collate results from various forms of treatment.

Consequently, I got the impression that the experts themselves were unsure about effective treatment. However, Dr Leyton took the conventional view that various kinds of chemotherapy should be effective, and would provide a life expectancy of about three years if I responded as expected. Without any chemotherapy, she thought I might only have a year or so left. The report made depressing reading, but from the legal point of view it emphasised the seriousness of the situation. Bentham had been concerned about how I would react to it, and rather than sending me a copy in the post, he had asked Mike and me to come to his office so that he could run through it with us. He did his best to emphasise that the report could well verge on the side of pessimism as this would help our case.

He was, in fact, worrying unnecessarily. I had already had similar, although slightly more optimistic news from Prof Greenwood, so the Leyton report came as no great shock. I therefore took the news quite calmly. Another reason for my equanimity was that I didn't entirely believe the report. It had always been my belief that the cancer threat had been 'sexed up' to cover up areas of negligence. Once this had been done –almost certainly by Ellman at Casterbridge Hospital – it had been perpetuated elsewhere. I had ovarian cancer – end of matter. No one, not even Prof Shaw, seemed particularly interested in investigating whether I had other problems as well, or even instead of cancer. There was some evidence, I felt, that this could indeed be the case. Prof Shaw had always believed my cancer was 'indolent' which suggested that some other process could be causing the formation of masses. Terry Sutton's subtle diagnostic techniques had never detected obvious signs of cancer, although I did show low resistance to it. The possibility that cancer could be the least of my worries wasn't entirely unrealistic.

Prof Greenwood's letter to Titchmouth Hospital following my private consultation with him, was a report of sorts. It agreed almost entirely with Dr Leyton's report regarding prognosis and treatment. Obviously, Bentham was keeping very quiet about the fact that during a phone conversation with Greenwood he had questioned the causative link, suggesting that in 2001 my disease was already so advanced that earlier referral would have made no difference. To some extent this remark confirmed what I had already suspected – Greenwood had not got a firm grasp of my medical history. Muir, on the other hand, who had spent many well-paid hours pouring over my notes, had reached a different conclusion.

These three reports had all been generated from my side. The defence had declined the right to produce a report to refute the causative link, which was why Bentham was so furious when it was found that Professor Heather Terry's report dealt with this issue, instead of addressing matters of treatment and prognosis, where, of course, the defence had the right to refute our reports if they could find an expert to do so. Bentham wrote a very firm letter to Vera Stone on the issue, threatening to raise the matter with the judge unless certain parts of the Terry report were withdrawn. It seemed that because the trial date was now less than a month away, and just about every oncology expert was now on holiday, the defence would not have their own report on treatment and prognosis.

However, by some miracle, everyone got their heads together, and before people departed for various exotic climes, a telephone conference between Muir, Leyton, and Terry was set up. Fortunately there was general agreement that I would need increasingly strong courses of chemotherapy, and that I could reasonably expect to live a further three years. Bentham asked me to write a letter to him outlining my thoughts on hearing this news. It obviously had to be a real sob-story, as this would help to push up the damages. My principal theme was that Mike and I had worked hard all our lives for a comfortable and active retirement to include travel, and activities and voluntary work in the community. I could no longer risk travel outside the EU because of health insurance problems. I could not take as active a role as I would like to in the community because I was now unreliable healthwise, and all I had to look forward to was three years of poor health dominated by increasingly debilitating courses of chemotherapy. I added that it was particularly distressing to know that Mike would be alone in old age, when, because I was ten years younger, I had fully expected to outlive him. I mentioned his own poor health, and that he had never been very practical, emphasising that he would need a lot of household help in my absence.

Bentham had warned me that if the case went to court I would have to be prepared to read out this letter in front of the judge. I very much hoped it wouldn't be necessary because basically I didn't believe a word of it. Acting had never been my strong point, and I very seldom lied even on minor issues because I felt everyone would sus me. I doubted whether I'd be able to inject sufficient emotion into the statement for it to be fully effective. The judge might smell a rat, and might come out with some comment like, "Mrs Bland, I'm not convinced that you truly believe what you are telling me. Are you holding back on something?" But isn't that what I really wanted? If I wanted truth and justice, my case, as it stood at present, would have to collapse. Unless it could then be reconstructed in a different form, Carr and Bentham would both lose an awful lot of income, and I wouldn't get anything, so would be seriously out of pocket. Things had to proceed as planned, and hopefully would be settled before the trial date.

On the 5th of August, which was between my stays in Titchmouth Hospital, Bentham, Mike and I went to Carr's chambers in London to finalise the details of the claim for damages.

"The purpose of this meeting is principally to discuss quantum," Carr announced.

"What's 'quantum'?" I asked.

"Who didn't pay attention in their Latin lessons!" Mike jeered. He was right. During most of my Latin lessons at grammar school I had played chess with my friend on a pocket set we passed between each other under the desk – something I had never regretted. After all, I'd got through nearly sixty years of life without the need for Latin, whereas chess had given me many hours of pleasure. Even now, faced with Latin legal terms, I had nice people to translate for me.

"Money, your damages," Bentham explained. For such a money-driven profession, lawyers seem remarkably reticent about actually mentioning the filthy lucre. They would just about manage to utter the word 'fees' in slightly strangulated tones, which was a good thing, because if Bentham had ever asked me for a 'consideration', I'd have considered it, but....

However, all reticence was soon abandoned as we got down to working out my 'quantum'. Firstly there was the general compensation for a permanent colostomy which was laid down in a booklet, but adjusted downwards for my age. Then there were the special damages – my out of pocket expenses such as travel to medical appointments and household help. On top of this we added anticipated future expenses such as private treatment I might need, and all the household help Mike would need to replace my services if I died. This last heading was, in fact, the largest item in the special damages. We spent hours tapping calculators and doing strange things with 'multipliers'. Finally we arrived at a figure of £184,000, which didn't surprise me, as a few weeks previously I had managed by myself to push the figure to nearly £200,000.

On reviewing the figures, it was very clear that the final amount was so high because of the household services for Mike if I died way before my time. It had to be based on his expected life span which would need to be properly assessed by an expert. Bentham was instructed to arrange this, as Carr was certain that the defence could dispute this heading.

"I think an out-of-court settlement is likely so long as we're seen to be flexible and reasonable," Carr concluded. He turned to Bentham. "Do you think we should ask for £150,000 in full and final settlement?"

"That would seem reasonable," Bentham concurred.

"What do you feel about that, Mrs Bland?" Carr asked me.

"I'd be more than happy with £150,000," I replied. "It's more than I thought I'd get." What the hell would I do with it all, I wondered.

"I don't think they'll agree to £150,000 though," Bentham cautioned. "I think £130,000 is more likely, and quite frankly, if that's the kind of offer we get, it might be wise to accept it. You see, if we held out for more, but then we didn't get it, you could be liable for some of their costs." He went into a great rigmarole about who was responsible for what costs in such a situation.

"I'd be happy with anything over £100,000," I said.

"What's your view on the matter, Mr Bland?" Carr asked. "You've been sitting there very quietly."

"I'd agree with Monica. I don't think it would be worth dragging things on for perhaps the odd few thousand."

It was therefore agreed that we should offer to settle for £150,000 and back it with the itemised quantum report amounting to £184,000. As we treated ourselves to a taxi back to Victoria Coach Station, we felt things had gone quite well. It really did seem that at last we were on the verge of a settlement.

We were now well into the holiday season and both Bentham and Carr were going to be away throughout the second half of August, just when we expected the other side to come up with an offer. Bentham thoroughly briefed one of his colleagues, a Mr Dodds, so that he could deal with any developments, and then departed with his family to Cornwall. It was now just a question of waiting.

On the 23rd of August I had an appointment at the cancer centre at Titchmouth. I was due to see Dr Merton, and I was fully expecting to have my first dose of chemotherapy. Knowing how much waiting around there would be, I went fully prepared with sandwiches, a banana, and plenty of reading matter. Dr Merton appeared satisfied that the stents were working well, and that therefore my renal system would be able to cope with the toxic chemotherapy. It appeared that he was about to write out the first recipe for the lab when a thought struck me.

"What was my most recent CA125 reading?" I asked. I'd had this blood test during my last visit for stent fitting, but hadn't had the result.

Dr Merton tapped a few keys on the computer and stared at the screen. "120," he replied.

"It's gone down then," I said. "In June it was 156."

He frowned, and tapped some more keys. "Yes, you're right." He looked totally confused. This wasn't meant to happen. My CA125 had been slowly rising for over a year, and as the cancer gradually took hold again, it was expected to go on rising. The chemo would probably reduce it, and the extent to which it fell would indicate the effectiveness of the treatment. However, I knew that CA125 readings were both complicated and inconclusive. 120 was still well above normal, but doctors had already told me that it was the rise and fall which was of more significance than the actual reading.

"That's quite a significant fall," Dr Merton went on. He appeared deep in thought, but offered no explanation. "I think it might be best to hold off the chemo for a while. We'll see how things are after your next CT scan."

I breathed a sigh of relief. With general confusion prevailing all around, appointments were made for my next scan in September, followed by a consultation. I then had to have kidney function tests to ensure that the stents were still working OK. I didn't get away from the hospital until three o'clock, so the sandwiches and reading matter came in useful after all.

As I walked back to the car, I got on the mobile to Mike.

"My CA125's down," I said. "They're not going to do chemo after all."

"That's good news."

"But why is it down? It seems to me it might not have been cancer that was raising it in the first place. Perhaps it was my poor kidney function, so the stenting has made it go down."

"That seems possible."

"You know, if I hadn't asked Merton what the most recent CA125 was, and then pointed out that it had fallen, I don't think he'd have noticed. I can't say I've got much faith in him. It seems I've escaped chemo by the skin of my teeth."

"Did he say he wasn't sure about the cancer or anything?"

"No. He didn't have any explanation for the fall, and I didn't ask. He's just booked me for another scan in September and then he'll review the situation. Tell you what, we'd better keep quiet about this. We don't want doubt about my condition at this late stage, do we? Hopefully the other side won't get to hear."

"But things are still very inconclusive it seems."

"Of course, but the other side will latch on to anything, won't they?"

"I can't see they'll find out before making an offer."

By now I had reached the car, parked in a back street to avoid the highway robbery the hospital called parking charges. I ended the call, saying I'd be home in under an hour. As I sped back along the motorway, I reflected on the unexpected news. I wasn't entirely surprised by it because it confirmed what continued to be my deeply-held belief – the cancer, if present at all, wasn't as serious as all the experts seemed to think. Previous ups and downs in my CA125 had indicated that other factors were at work, and at this particular time my poorly functioning kidneys were probably largely to blame. However, I also knew that some cancer did not cause a rise in CA125. It seemed that this test was so inconclusive and misleading that it was surprising the doctors bothered to do it.

I turned my mind to the legal aspect. Merton had been contacted by Bentham at some stage and therefore knew about my case. He could alert someone concerned with the defence to the latest development. But would he? That would take time. It was quite possible that virtually everyone connected with the case was now on holiday. There was only two weeks to go to the trial date. For all I knew, the defence had already got an offer for settlement in the pipeline. In the circumstances, was it morally correct for me to keep quiet about the latest development? After all, it was inconclusive, and therefore might not be regarded as significant by the experts. It would delay everything while yet more medical opinion was sought. The trial would be delayed, throwing the court into confusion. Meanwhile all the lawyers would be making yet more money which would all have to be met by the medical insurers. At the end of it all, the outcome might be pretty much the same. Looked at in that way, it struck me that the moral course was indeed to keep quiet.

Between phoning Mike and arriving home, a fax had arrived from Dodds consisting of a letter from Burnham Brown with a final offer of £100,000. It was rather less than I had been led to expect, but the letter was full of threats about the arguments they would use if the trial proceeded. It seemed they were planning to use Prof Terry for evidence in court. She was the expert who questioned the causative link. It was her belief that I would be in my present condition even if Foyle had referred me to a new consultant in 2001. My own experts, Muir and Leyton, disagreed with her. Although my legal advisers doubted whether any aspect of causation could be raised at this stage, I felt that Prof Terry could cause problems. The judge would take notice of one of the most eminent experts in the field, and this might lead him to question wider aspects of the case, and open the can of worms which I still believed was deeply buried somewhere. But isn't this what I wanted? It was, but the consequences could now be horrendous. My entire case, in its present form, could collapse, and I would be responsible for the legal fees of the defence. In other words, I could lose, rather than gain, £100,000, and that would leave me little more than my meagre pensions to live on. It was too great a risk.

Another point raised by Burnham Brown was that I had no legal right to claim for the loss Mike would suffer if I was no longer able to care for him. They quoted some case law on the matter which meant very little to me, but as such a substantial part of my special damages was for this provision, it was an important point.

While I was trying to make sense of it all, and realising that I only had until four o'clock on the 25th to accept or reject the offer, a fax arrived from Mr Dodds. In it he suggested that much of the threatened court activity was probably bluff, but he admitted that he was uncertain about the validity of the point about Mike's losses. He was urgently seeking expert opinion from a barrister. Should he rule in favour of the defence, Mr Dodds suggested I should accept the £100,000. He explained that if the case came to trial, and I did not get a better offer, I would be liable for the defence's costs from the time the offer was made. In other words, I could end up with less.

The situation was very confusing, and it was very unfortunate that both Bentham and Carr were on holiday. Dodds was obviously doing a good job, but he didn't have such a thorough knowledge of my case as the other two. That evening I faxed a letter back to Dodds agreeing with him that I thought the threats were bluff, and that so long as it was ruled I could claim for Mike's losses, we should hold out in the hope that the offer would be upped before the trial. The tone was rather more gung-ho than I actually felt.

The next day, the 24th, Dodds faxed me details of a case

which supported the defence's argument about claiming for Mike's care. It seemed that they did indeed have a point. We should have included Mike in the action, but, of course, at the time the case had started, it was far from obvious that my life was at risk. Things had changed so much since my initial meeting with Bentham in November 2002, nearly three years ago. Nothing more happened that day because we were waiting for the opinion of the barrister.

During the small hours of the 25th I woke up with everything circulating round in my head. I think I had been dreaming I was in court and that everything was going wrong. I tossed and turned as my over-active brain ran through various scenarios. If the case went to court, the defence had every right to see the very latest medical notes, as did my own team. The falling CA125 would set alarm bells ringing everywhere. Bentham and Carr would be on at me – "How long have you known about this? You should have told us immediately." All the experts would want the opportunity to review their reports. At very best, I might only get some interim award for the colostomy, while the cancer situation was clarified. I certainly wouldn't get £100,000, and therefore would probably be liable for some of the defence's costs. The judge would take a jaundiced view of everyone – incompetent expert witnesses and a deceitful plaintif. It just didn't bear thinking about.

Next morning over the breakfast table, I discussed things with Mike.

"I've been thinking," I announced.

"Oh yeah?" It was said in his usual tone which implied I was incapable of rational thought.

"I think I must accept this £100,000."

"I've been thinking that too. I think if you went to court you could end up with less, and in the light of the latest developments the case could even collapse. I don't think you'd exactly be flavour of the month with Bentham and Carr if that happened."

"Exactly. I reckon they'd have kittens if I told them about the latest CA125 result."

"It's time to take the money and call it a day. After all, you've done much better than you expected to. When you started this case you thought you'd get about ten to fifteen thousand for an unnecessary operation."

"True, but look what I've been through since. I don't think the award is excessive."

"So are you going to phone Dodds and tell him your decision?"

"I'll wait until he sends the barrister's opinion, which should be this morning. Then even if it's in our favour, which I doubt, I'll fax him a letter accepting the £100,000. He'll get it to Burnham Brown before the four o'clock deadline."

Later that morning the barrister's opinion was faxed to me, and, as expected, it sided with the defence. I immediately wrote a short letter to Dodds accepting the offer of £100,000 plus my costs. As it whirred through the fax machine I felt a great sense of relief. After nearly five years of battling, it was all over. Things had not worked out as I would have wished. I still didn't really know what had been going on in my pelvis, and as far as I was aware, no doctors had been disciplined, although Foyle must have been ruing the error of his ways. But I had the satisfaction of knowing I had done everything I could have done, and that the financial outcome was better than I had expected.

CHAPTER 30

It was now just a question of dotting the Is and crossing the Ts. I didn't actually get my £100,000 until the 30th of September. I immediately took £20,000 for myself which was to cover the legal costs I had incurred in the abortive action against Casterbridge Hospital, the genuine expense of travel and private treatment to date, and a bit more to reward myself for all the hours spent dealing with the case. The remaining £80,000 went into a building society. The interest would be nearly £4,000 a year which I thought would be enough to cover my health-related expenses. The capital would only be drawn down if I needed treatment not available on the NHS, or if Mike needed a lot of household help if I died or became permanently incapacitated. Any funds remaining on Mike's death would go to Cancer Research UK. To some extent I didn't regard the money as mine to fritter away. It had been awarded to me for a specific purpose, and if it was not needed for that purpose, it was only right that it should be returned to the medical world. At least I had the satisfaction of being able to direct the funds to where I felt they were needed. I redrafted my will to make my wishes clear.

Bentham put in a claim for his costs. It came to a few thousand more than my settlement, which didn't surprise me. Being on a conditional fee agreement, both Bentham and Carr had done very well out of me. However, the claim had to be approved by some independent body, and it was adjusted downwards to a few thousand less than my settlement. I got a little back to cover fees I had paid before I was put on the conditional fee agreement. However, £900 of what was due was withheld for a year in case we had to pay Jessop for his useless report. Fortunately he let the matter drop, and the money was eventually paid to me.

At some stage I must have verbally told Bentham about the falling CA125 resulting in me not having more chemo for the time being, as one of his letters refers to my 'good news'. It was a matter we all wanted to keep rather quiet about.

I had hoped that now I would be able to 'move on' as they say. But when you're lumbered with a malfunctioning body, forever throwing up unexpected things, that just isn't possible. My thoughts were seldom very far from my pelvis. Just what was going on? The doctors didn't seem to know, and I certainly didn't.

It seemed I would always need stents in my ureters, and these had to be changed every six months, which meant a brief visit to hospital. I was adamant that I was not going to suffer again from the terrible pain I had experienced when they were put in, so I asked that the procedure be done under general anaesthetic. For some reason Titchmouth Hospital just didn't do this, saying general anaesthetic wasn't necessary. Anyway, they referred me back to Sandcliffe Hospital, which was more convenient for me, and where they always used anaesthetic for stent changes. It was amazing that two hospitals should have such different methods.

The stents had been causing constant urinary infections throughout the autumn of 2005. I was practically living on antibiotics, and it made me wonder whether the stents were inserted properly, given the unexpected pain I had endured during the procedure. Then just after Christmas 2005 I was rushed into Casterbridge A and E with severe rectal bleeding. I was passing great big clots every few minutes. It was absolutely terrifying, and nobody seemed to know what was causing it and what to do about it. After a few hours it stopped. I was not allowed to eat or drink in case an operation was needed, and I nearly died of thirst. After a few tests I was allowed home two days later, still no wiser as to what was happening. Twelve hours later, at five am, I was bleeding again. Mike called an ambulance. This time matters were taken more seriously. But it was now New Year's Eve, not the best of times to be admitted to hospital with an undiagnosed condition. The period between Christmas and New Year is like one very long week-end. Consultants like to have some time off, their juniors are likely to be hung over or busy anticipating the next party, and any routine the hospital has managed to establish has probably gone to pot. I guessed that nothing much would be done until Tuesday the 3rd of January when things would slowly return to normal.

However, I had now lost a lot of blood and was therefore transfused with four units which made me feel a little better. The bleeding stopped again, but still nobody seemed to know what had caused it. A junior doctor asked me what I thought had caused it, and the only thing I could think of was something wrong with the stents, causing internal injury. These now needed replacing, but Sandcliffe Hospital had yet to make the arrangements. The Casterbridge doctors decided to contact Dr Merton at Titchmouth, seeing he was the consultant I was officially under at the time, and this led to me having another CT scan. Nobody told me what this showed, but on the 6th of January, within hours of the result becoming available to the doctors, I was transferred to the urology ward at Sandcliffe Hospital. It did indeed seem there was a problem with the stents, although no one told me exactly what. I had a degree of renal failure, which explained my occasional bouts of sickness. I was a bit of an emergency and that evening a nephrotomy tube was put into my left kidney. Within hours I started to feel better. I had my own room at Sandcliffe, a precautionary regulation because I had been transferred from another hospital. I certainly wasn't complaining about that.

Before leaving Casterbridge Hospital I had seen a Dr Sarah Dixon, a radiologist. She explained that she thought the bleeding had been caused by the tumour pressing on and rupturing a blood vessel. It seemed feasible.

"We can try and shrink the tumour with radiotherapy," she said.

"But I've been told I can't have radiotherapy because I've had it before, and it wouldn't do any good anyway."

"I've dug out your old records," Dr Dixon explained. "You only had a mild dose back in '81, and that was twenty-five years ago. Your body can easily take a further dose. I would recommend that you have ten sessions on a daily basis. Modern radiotherapy is very accurate and focused. We can direct it right at the tumour. I think it would be the best treatment for you."

This really was a turn-up. All the top experts, and, indeed, all the research literature, no longer rated radiotherapy as an effective treatment for ovarian cancer. Yet here was this Dr Dixon, whom I'd never met before, recommending it. Because she had gone to the trouble of finding my old records, she had quite obviously given my case some thought.

"But will it do any good? I've been led to believe it wouldn't," I said.

"I think it would be very beneficial for your condition," Dr Dixon assured me.

'Your condition'. I pondered the words. Why hadn't she said 'your cancer'? Dr Dixon treated cancer all the time. She wasn't afraid of the word, and she knew I'd lived with the threat of cancer long enough not to get all funny about it myself. Radiotherapy was used to treat all kinds of growth and tumours, not just malignant ones. There was no denying I had some kind of tumour, but was it malignant?

I agreed to the radiotherapy, and because my legal action (which could always have swung back on to Casterbridge Hospital) was now concluded, I agreed that my further treatment should now be conducted entirely in Casterbridge. It was a drag going to Titchmouth, and I'd never had much faith in Dr Merton.

I had new stents fitted on the 12th of January. The nef tube remained in place but clamped off so that the efficiency of the new stents could be assessed. They appeared not to be working very well, and I started to feel sick again. My creatin levels rose. The tube was unclamped and I was told that it would have to remain in place until well after the radiotherapy was over. Apparently they thought the treatment might cause more swelling in my pelvis, and they wanted to ensure that I didn't suffer renal failure again.

I was still in Sandcliffe Hospital when I was due for my pre-radiotherapy checks by Dr Dixon at Casterbridge on the 16th of January. Unfortunately urology was only dealt with at Sandcliffe, and radiotherapy was only done at Casterbridge. It was up to Sandcliffe to arrange transport for my ten o'clock appointment at Casterbridge. The two hospitals were only about eight miles apart and the journey took about twenty minutes. I was told I would be taken by taxi, and that a porter would take me down to reception. By nine thirty I was ready and waiting, but nothing happened. At nine forty-five I pointed out to the ward staff that I would be late for my appointment. I was rebuked for complaining, and told that Casterbridge knew I'd be arriving a little late.

I finally got to Casterbridge Hospital at three o'clock. It was quite obvious that someone had forgotten to order the transport but hadn't admitted it. I began to feel that Sandcliffe urology department couldn't organise a booze-up in a brewery, and I had no idea how I would ever get to my radiotherapy sessions on time. Fortunately I was still able to see Dr Dixon.

"Well, you've been leading us a merry dance," she greeted me, as if my lateness was all my fault. Perhaps it was a good thing that words completely failed me, because anything I might have uttered wouldn't have been fit for her ears. She wanted to start radiotherapy in two days' time, so I concluded that I just had to get myself discharged from Sandcliffe. Fortunately, when I saw the doctors the following morning they agreed that the practice nurse at my GP's surgery could look after the nef tube, and that I was well enough to drive myself from home to my radiotherapy sessions.

So, once again, after twenty five years. I was back on the narrow stretcher under the massive radiotherapy machine. I was told the treatment was more accurate and sophisticated these days, but the delivery method didn't seem to have changed at all. Beams of light and indelible marks on my abdomen had to be lined up, and then I was zapped briefly from above and below. I had a session on my sixtieth birthday, the 30th of January, and although I had to give my date of birth every day as an identity check, the nurses didn't even notice.

"Thirty, one, forty-six," I said with great emphasis and a smile. No response, the miserable buggers.

When I'd had my ten sessions Dr Dixon said she was handing me over to Dr Oswald. I felt I had come full circle. I remained suspicious of Dr Oswald, although I had the feeling he had quite genuinely been misled by Ellman. But it had been Dr Oswald who had referred me to Prof Shaw, so in some ways I felt grateful towards him.

At the beginning of April I went back to Sandcliffe Hospital to have new stents fitted. As usual, the urology department appeared to be in a state of chaos. At six o'clock in the morning the day after I had been admitted I was told to get ready to go to theatre because I was top of the list. I pointed out that I had not seen a doctor since coming in, and that I had not yet signed a consent form. A junior doctor hurriedly thrust one into my hands, but I refused to sign it until I had discussed exactly what they intended to do. Meanwhile I was made to put on one of those hideous open-back gowns they make you wear for operations. Then a few minutes later a rather more senior doctor appeared.

"I'm afraid we won't be operating on you today," he said. "You're not on the list."

I was furious. "How can I be on top of the list one minute, and not even on it the next? Someone's been lying to me." I spoke loudly, making sure the whole six-bed room could hear.

The doctor didn't have anything to say about it.

"We'll clamp off the nef tube to see if the existing stents can cope," he said. "Then we'll have you in again for a stent change."

Later on a senior nurse came and apologised about the mix-up, and provided a rather unconvincing explanation about why it had happened. For about the first time ever, they had actually admitted to a mistake. It seemed that all the staff on the ward had now heard about it, including Tom, the tea boy (a middle-aged man actually). What with my frequent visits to the ward, we had become quite friendly and we always had a little chat as he served my coffee and biscuits.

"That mix-up this morning must have been a bit upsetting," he commented sympathetically.

"Yes," I agreed. "Things like that shouldn't happen. It makes you wonder what goes on that you don't even know about."

"Exactly," he replied with a dark look. Like me, Tom had a pretty jaundiced view of the ward organisation, and probably knew of far worse episodes than what had happened to me.

"Mind you," I went on, "bearing in mind things that have happened to me in the past, it's not that awful. That's why I'm not getting too uptight about it."

"Really?" Tom seemed to want to know more, but there wasn't time to launch into my medical and litigation history.

"Oh yes! I could write a book about it."

"Why don't you?"

We both smiled as he pushed his trolley off to the next

bed, but later that day I dressed and strolled along to the near by Tesco superstore. It was nice to leave the hospital for a few minutes and get back into the normal, familiar world. I bought a big thick A4 notepad, and that afternoon I started my book. It was a story that had to be told.

Next day Tom saw me scribbling away.

"I've started a book," I told him.

"Wow! Put me down for a copy when it's published."

"Huh!" I had no illusions about the likelihood of getting it published unless I chose to do it myself.

The clamping off of the nef tube indicated that the existing stents were working OK, so the tube was removed and I was discharged at the end of the week. The stents were replaced in May without incident.

On the 21st of April I had a consultation with Dr Oswald at Casterbridge Hospital. As I sat down he indicated a small dictaphone on his desk.

"Because of the trouble in the past, I'd like to record this meeting," he explained. "Is that all right with you?"

"Yes, but I'd like a copy please."

"I'll see what I can do."

I couldn't really complain. Hadn't I secretly recorded my meeting with Harcourt back in 2002? At least he was being open about it. However, it was unusual, and it strongly suggested to me that some kind of wrong-doing had occurred in the past, and that Oswald had found himself inadvertently dragged into it. He now wanted to be squeaky clean, and the recording was for his own protection.

"So, what's been going on since your operation at the City and Royal?"

I told him about my chemotherapy at Titchmouth, my stent problems at Sandcliffe, the rectal bleeding, and my occasional vaginal infections which were being ineffectively treated by my GP.

"What do you understand are the reasons for the rectal bleeding?"

"Well, I can only tell you what Dr Dixon told me – that the tumour had ruptured a blood vessel."

He didn't comment. "I think the way forward is to keep you closely monitored. We'll have another CT scan in June and we'll keep an eye on your CA125."

"How reliable is the CA125 test?"

"Not very, as it's not only cancer that causes it to rise. But a rise is an indication that we need to investigate further. Combined with the results of the scan, it can be useful."

Arrangements were made for future tests and scans. As I left I realised I had done nearly all the talking. If anything inaccurate about my diagnoses or treatment had been uttered, it would have come from me – either from my own head, or from what other doctors had told me. In other words, if there was anything wrong, it hadn't come from Oswald, and he could prove it with the recording. Once bitten, twice shy, I thought. It was yet further confirmation of my long-held beliefs. I never got a copy of the recording, but that didn't concern me.

The CT scan in June showed that the tumour had decreased in size, indicating that the radiotherapy had had some beneficial effect. The CA125 was 15, completely normal.

"I don't think we'll bother with any more CA125 tests," Oswald announced. "It seems your sort of cancer doesn't cause a rise – not all do."

So, he was still making the assumption that I had active cancer. He could equally well have concluded that the CA125 was normal because I didn't have cancer. Had all the fluctuations in my CA125 been entirely due to something else? If so, what was that something else? It seemed there was very little joined-up thinking on my case, and everything was still clouded by the mysteries of my past history. There could be no 'moving on', and the dictaphone was still on the desk.

I continued to see Oswald at four month intervals, with CT scans about every six months. In January 2007 I was told the tumour had not grown, suggesting the cancer was dormant.

"If you doctors are to be believed," I said, "I've had ovarian cancer for twenty-six years. Why aren't I dead?"

Oswald looked uncomfortable. The dictaphone was no longer on the desk. "I think Prof Shaw did a very good job," he said. "And it's also due to your type of cancer, a very slowly developing one."

It was difficult to believe this second point, especially as Terry Sutton was increasingly convinced that I had no sign of cancer at the present time. Another appointment was made for May. There was to be no scan in the meantime, and Dr Oswald never made any physical examinations at his consultations. It seemed he was relying on me to detect any abnormalities in my condition, but seeing I hadn't been told to look out for any specific problem, I was somewhat in the dark. Everyone feels a bit off now and again and odd little aches and pains are not unusual, especially as you get older. It would be stupid for me to panic about every little twinge, but how could I tell what was serious?

I had told Oswald about a problem with my recent stent change at Sandcliffe when they were not sure if one of the new stents was fitted correctly. They had left the other one in, but this was now well overdue for replacement. Friends had been telling me that I didn't look well, and I had to admit that I felt tired, sometimes breathless, and lacking energy, although not really ill. I think Oswald could tell that there was indeed something wrong with me because he ordered an urgent blood test before I left the hospital.

That afternoon he phoned me with the result.

"Your kidney function is very poor," he said. "I've made arrangements for you to be admitted to Sandcliffe Hospital immediately. Can you get yourself over to A and E in the next hour or so?"

"Goodness! Is it that urgent? I feel OK."

"It's important you get treatment as soon as possible. Otherwise there could be permanent kidney damage."

I packed a bag and took the direct bus to Sandcliffe Hospital, reporting to A and E about an hour later. I saw my name being written up on a whiteboard – Monica Bland – renal failure. It seemed I was indeed an emergency. Once again I had Dr Oswald to thank for getting me the attention I needed, and unlike when he had referred me to Prof Shaw, this time he had acted quickly.

But the Sandcliffe A and E department was in its usual state of total chaos, and it was many hours before I was moved to a ward and put under the care of a urologist. I suspected that this latest crisis was entirely due to a combination of poor treatment and complete lack of follow-up. I felt extremely annoyed. Had it not been for my check-up with Oswald, I might have suffered permanent renal failure. I could sue them, I thought, but rapidly decided against it. What good would it do?

The following morning, a Saturday, a nephrotomy tube was put into my left kidney. I was soon passing considerably more than I was taking in both orally and via a drip. It seemed my recent slight weight gain had been due to fluid retention, not over-indulgence at Christmas. In fact, when I eventually got home and weighed myself, I found I had lost eleven pounds in ten days. It seemed I was much iller than I had thought because over the next few days I had intravenous antibiotics and four units of blood because it was found I was seriously anaemic.

As usual, the general care was chaotic. I was moved three times in a week. This was because the enormous urology department was ninety per cent male, so the few females had to be gathered together in whatever sized bed bay was suitable for their number. Briefly, I was the only woman, and therefore had a side room. Unfortunately I was there for less than a day. Poor Tom, the tea boy, never knew where he'd find me next. Then I was put in a bay not equipped with the Patientline TVs. The other patients were so gaga they didn't need TV, but I did. I was furious, and as I was feeling better and not actually receiving any treatment, I discharged myself for a few days until they were ready to fit new stents.

Because of the problem previously with the right stent, it was decided that this should be inserted via the kidney rather than via the bladder. This is how it had been done at Titchmouth, and in this case it was indeed normal to do it without general anaesthetic. I was dreading it, and told the doctors about the pain I had experienced before. As had been the case at Titchmouth, they seemed surprised. But this time I only had a certain amount of discomfort, suggesting that the procedure had not been done properly at Titchmouth.

My general health now improved. Then in March, without any warning, I had another heavy bleed, from the vagina this time. I woke up in the small hours with blood pouring out of me. Mike called an ambulance and I was rushed into Casterbridge A and E, and, as before, left lying on a trolley for hours, bleeding to death, or so I thought. But my vital signs were stable. It seemed I wasn't in any danger. The blood was mainly in the form of large clots, as if it had been accumulating for some time and had now found a way out. But where had it come from?

I was eventually taken to the gynae ward.

"Don't put me under Ellman," I told the junior doctor who was looking after me. "He and I have fallen out in the past. Put me under Harcourt because he was the last gynaecologist I saw in 2002."

It was decided that this was the most sensible course of action. Amazingly, I was given a room to myself. Was it just a lucky coincidence, or was it to ensure that Ellman and I didn't catch sight of each other? Or was it because the reputation I was building up at Sandcliffe had preceded me to Casterbridge? The hospital authorities had probably decided I was trouble. I made sure other patients on the ward knew when cock-ups occurred. I had been heard dispensing legal advice, bragging about my successful litigation, trying to convince patients that they could sue for negligence, and recommending an excellent chap at Jeffreys and Rowe. I was fairly sure that such behaviour had got me an early discharge from the urology hell-hole. If you're in a single room you have very little contact with other patients.

I was given two units of blood, and kept under observation for three days. The bleeding had stopped after a few hours, as before. I never saw a consultant, but was told there was to be a multi-disciplinary meeting about me. Someone would phone me to discuss the conclusion. I was surprised no kind of X-ray or scan was done to try and detect the reason for the bleeding.

I heard nothing. It confirmed my increasingly strongly held belief – the doctors didn't have a clue what was going on in my pelvis, and they didn't want to find out. Perhaps they were scared I might find a reason to sue them for wrong diagnosis, unnecessary treatments, and the like. Or perhaps it would mean they would have to come clean about what had happened in the past. Then there would be an awful lot of red faces.

I had won my case, I had eighty thousand pounds in my designated health fund account in a building society, I was usually fairly well, but I was in limbo, and that is where I was going to remain. Viv, my hairdresser, could look forward to many future episodes of the on-going real life soap opera.